THE REAL COST OF FRACKING

THE REAL COST
OF FRACKING

How America's Shale Gas Boom
Is Threatening Our Families,
Pets, and Food

MICHELLE BAMBERGER
and ROBERT OSWALD

Foreword by **SANDRA STEINGRABER**

BEACON PRESS
BOSTON

Beacon Press books
are published under the auspices of
the Unitarian Universalist Association of Congregations.

17 16 15 14   8 7 6 5 4 3 2 1

This book is printed on acid-free paper that meets the uncoated paper
ANSI/NISO specifications for permanence as revised in 1992.

Text design and composition by Wilsted & Taylor Publishing Services

The names and other identifying characteristics of many people
mentioned in this book have been changed to protect their identities.

LIBRARY OF CONGRESS CATALOGING-IN-PUBLICATION DATA
Bamberger, Michelle.
  The real cost of fracking : how America's shale-gas boom is threatening our families,
pets, and food / Michelle Bamberger and Robert Oswald ; foreword by Sandra
Steingraber.
     pages cm
  Includes bibliographical references and index.
  ISBN 978-0-8070-8493-9 (hardcover : alk. paper)—ISBN 978-0-8070-8494-6 (ebook)
  1. Hydraulic fracturing—Environmental aspects—United States. 2. Shale gas industry
—Environmental aspects—United States. 3. Gas well drilling—Environmental aspects
—United States. 4. Pets—Effect of stress on. I. Oswald, Robert, 1953– II. Title.
  TD195.G3B36 2014
  363.17'91—dc23   2014000487

For the animals

CONTENTS

FOREWORD

Years ago, my home state of Illinois entertained the proposals of an industry that claimed to have a magic solution to both fossil fuel dependency and overflowing landfills: generate electricity by burning garbage, including industrial waste.

Thus began the incinerator wars.

In the early 1990s, one such facility was sited a half mile from my grandfather's farm. Members of the village board that green-lighted its application were wined and dined by the out-of-state owners and enticed by promises of a new school library. Some of them, as it turned out, were also investors with a direct financial stake in the outcome.

On the other side were farmers who stood to lose their water, their property values, the peaceful enjoyment of their homes, and the privilege of piloting their tractors down county roads unclogged with convoys of trucks ferrying toxic ash.

Tensions were high. Neighbors squared off against neighbors; opinions within families splintered; brothers were no longer on speaking terms. And yet, public conversation about the issue roiling the community was, at first, rare. When I asked my grandmother why her church did not take a position on the incinerator, her reply came in the form of a truism:

Silence is the sound of money talking.

Two decades later, there are no trash incinerators in downstate Illinois. A forceful citizen uprising eventually put an end to all nine proposed incinerators, and nary a one was built. (Which is a very good outcome. What was then called "state of the art" would be, by now—as municipalities in other states went on to discover—dangerous, fire-breathing relics and a sunk-cost disincentive to curbside recycling.)

It was data that broke the silence. The data said that incinerators, even state-of-the-art ones, emit a potent synthetic carcinogen: dioxin. While rural communities considered the seductive pitches from incinerator salesmen, the United States Environmental Protection Agency released a draft of its long-awaited dioxin reassessment; risk analyses were promulgated; and emissions data were published and publicized.

In response to the science, people started talking.

They said: Dioxin lasts in soil and in human fat for thirty-five to fifty years.

They said: Dioxin causes cancer, incinerators make dioxin, and, look, here are good studies to back up these facts.

They said: One overturned ash truck on a windy day spells ruin. And even without accidents, dioxin will seed itself into the air from the fly ash—and sift down over farm country, over the soil that is the beginning of the food chain, over our hogs and turkeys, over creation itself.

The message that science brought was transformational—especially when amplified by community teach-ins, ballot referenda, letters to the editor by local physicians, and a float in the annual Fourth of July parade that proclaimed, "God recycles, and the Devil burns." By the time all the talking reached the buyers of central Illinois' agricultural products (e.g., popcorn), a new day had dawned.

The incinerator wars at the end of the last century became the fracking wars at the beginning of this one. This time, however, science has been bound, gagged, and tossed into a corner.

At least three layers of scientific silence surround fracking.*

---

*Like the authors, I use the word *fracking* in an expansive way to refer to the entire unholy process of shale gas and oil extraction—from drilling and cementing a mile-deep, mile-long, L-shaped hole, to smashing apart bedrock with

Making up the first are legal exemptions—granted by the 2005 Energy Policy Act—to key provisions of our federal environmental statutes. These allow companies engaged in the extraction of gas and oil from shale via fracking to conceal the names of the chemicals and chemical mixtures they blast down holes in the ground. No other industry can withhold such information. Fracking companies are also unburdened by any requirement to monitor their emissions. Methane may seep out of well casings; heavy metals may slosh out of flowback pits; benzene may rise from wellheads and compressor stations; radon may be pushed through pipelines; formaldehyde may flow from flare stacks. But no one is routinely measuring it and estimating its cumulative impact.

And without right-to-know data or emissions data, public health science doesn't operate very well. Without knowing what chemicals and mixtures are used and what pollutants are released, researchers can't systematically measure human exposures or definitively connect exposures to health outcomes.

Second is the silence emanating from state and federal agencies, which both remain curiously uncurious about the public health effects of fracking.

With more than 6,000 active gas wells and more than 3,300 documented violations, Pennsylvania is already an intensely fracked state—with much more fracking to come. And yet neither the Pennsylvania Department of Environmental Protection nor the US EPA has conducted comprehensive measurements of air and water contaminants. And neither agency has made any systematic effort to interpret the findings they do possess. It was detective work by the *Scranton Times-Tribune* that found—buried deep in the Department of Environmental Protection's own records—161 cases of water contamination from fracking in Pennsylvania.[1] It was an individual engineering professor, slogging through industry statistics, who discovered just how leaky cement well casings really are: operator records show that the well casings of 6

---

prodigious amounts of water, sand, and chemicals to the conveyance of pressurized gas through pipelines, to the jet-roar of sixty-foot flare stacks, to the fleets of trucks ferrying fracking waste through residential areas.

to 7 percent of new gas wells drilled in Pennsylvania fail outright or
suffer from structural problems that could result in groundwater contamination.[2]

When it uncovered actual evidence of such contamination in real
people's drinking water, the US EPA bowed to industry pressure and
suspended all further investigation.

In Dimock, Pennsylvania.

In Pavillion, Wyoming.

In Weatherford, Texas.[3]

And, so, where there should be inquiry, debate, hearings, and peer-
review publications, there is only the sound of a closing book.

The third layer of silence takes the form of nondisclosure agreements and the hush money that comes with them. These take the form
of contracts with secrecy clauses that are signed by homeowners who
allege that their water has been ruined or their health damaged by
nearby drilling and fracking operations. In such cases, the price of a cash
settlement or property buy-out is the agreement *to tell no one* the story of
what happened—not the neighbors, not the newspapers, and not the
public health community. Ever.

A 2013 investigation by *Bloomberg News* of hundreds of regulatory
and legal filings across the nation found this kind of enforced silence to
be the rule rather than the exception. A strategy of muzzling accusations
of harm with sealed settlements, noted *Bloomberg* reporters, "keeps data
from regulators, policy makers, the news media and health researchers,
and makes it difficult to challenge the industry's claim that fracking has
never tainted anyone's water."[4]

In at least one case, the lifelong ban on speaking out about the harm
of fracking—imposed as part of a cash settlement—extended to all
members of a family, including young children. The Hallowich family
of southwestern Pennsylvania had claimed that drilling and fracking operations near their home had sickened them and damaged the value of
their property. Their agreement with the industry—including the dra-
conian family-wide gag order—came to light when the *Pittsburgh Post-
Gazette* itself successfully petitioned to unseal the court records. (Full
disclosure: Both the authors and I were among a group of scientists who
supported this petition as part of an amicus brief.)

In Pennsylvania, the code of enforced silence has even ensnared physicians. According to a state law called Act 13, doctors may obtain information from a gas drilling company about the specific identity of proprietary chemicals used in fracking operations to which their patients may have been exposed. In exchange for this confidential information, however, they must give up their right to warn the public —including patients and including public health authorities—about the health dangers associated with fracking. As I am writing, a federal judge has just denied a doctor in Pennsylvania the right to challenge in a lawsuit the constitutionality of Act 13.[5]

Against this background of the unspoken, the suppressed, the stifled, the gag-ordered, and the censored comes this important book. Ultimately, *The Real Cost of Fracking* is a collection of stories that bear witness to extremity. Its narrators, as the book's title implies, are the voices of real people living in the fracking fields of America. As these chapters make clear, they have endured conditions of corporate censorship, persecution, occupation, and virtual house arrest. Under the protection of pseudonyms, they are—in some cases for the first time—breaking silence and speaking out.

And because my fellow writers on the oil and gas industry's payroll will predictably attempt to dismiss these testimonies as "anecdotes," let me save us all a lot of time and say right now: Don't even bother.

The coauthors of this book—scientist and veterinarian—have done far more than assemble the words of human witnesses. They also translate for us a story that is inscribed in the bodies of animals—wildlife, livestock, pets—that live alongside the human narrators of this book. Here are the autopsy reports, the blood tests, the records of birth defects and reproductive outcomes, the air samples, the water-testing results. Here, woven among the courageous words of human witnesses, is the unimpeachable story of science carried out in extreme and intimidating circumstances.

It is the sound of silence breaking. It is speech to inspire our own. Let's pull up a chair and listen.

SANDRA STEINGRABER

INTRODUCTION

In the summer of 2009, we were awakened. Articles began to appear in our local papers on the subject of fracking, the common name for the entire process of unconventional gas extraction (horizontal drilling with high-volume hydraulic fracturing) whereby millions of gallons of water, sand, and chemicals are pushed deep into the earth under high pressure to release small pockets of gas held tightly in the rock (see "A Primer on Gas Drilling" in the appendix). In our tight-knit community, people on both sides of the issue enthusiastically expressed their opinions. One article in particular caught our attention and led us to a website[1] indicating that our small property in upstate New York was surrounded by neighbors who had already leased their lands to energy companies for gas drilling. We learned that our land could be drilled under and the gas extracted without our consent.[2] That is, as long as a gas company owns leases on at least a certain percentage of the land (in New York, it is 60 percent) inside a certain amount of space (typically, one square mile), gas can be extracted from properties within that area even if the company does not have a lease on that land. Unleased land is taken by a process known as *compulsory integration*.

We were concerned about what this meant for our water and air—as yet untainted—but we also wondered if our farmers' markets, CSAs (community-supported agriculture groups), and Finger Lakes wineries could survive the massive industrialization we were beginning to see in Pennsylvania. Would faculty, staff, and students—the mainstay of our economy—continue to be attracted to Cornell University and Ithaca College if the lakes and streams were polluted, the air fouled, and the land mottled by a matrix of shale gas wells? Would tourists continue to visit our picturesque parks, waterfalls, and gorges if thwarted by drilling traffic and diesel fumes?

Because of our interest in veterinary medicine, we became keenly aware of what was happening to companion animals and livestock in areas near existing industrial oil and gas operations. We heard stories we found hard to believe: healthy cattle dying within one hour after exposure to hydraulic fracturing fluid; cows failing to reproduce and herds with high rates of stillborn and stunted calves after exposure to drilling wastewater; dogs failing to reproduce after drinking contaminated well water; cats, dogs, and horses developing unexplained rashes and having difficulty breathing after living in intensively drilled areas. Our search for what really happened in each situation led us to document exposures and subsequent health problems by detailed case reports—just as would be done for a new disease[3]—in both animals and their owners.[4] We discovered that all too often, the humans in the household also experienced health problems associated with drilling operations and that sometimes the symptoms were the same ones their pets or farm animals had experienced.

As we soon learned, the potential threat to our community is just a small part of a worldwide debate that has at its core the values and essence of modern life. That is, we require energy to live in the modern world, but what degree of risk and environmental degradation are acceptable to obtain that energy? Who should be asked to sacrifice, and who should profit?

After untold hours of research, we learned more about the fossil fuel industry than we ever thought we'd have a reason to know. Drilling originally exploited pockets of oil or gas and, in most cases, had a small impact on the communities surrounding the drilling sites, as confirmed by many of the people we interviewed. The changes in recent years, which involve extracting gas directly from shales rather than pockets of gas, have been made possible by two technologies: horizontal drilling and hydraulic fracturing. Shale layers are 50 to 200 feet thick, and in order to contact more of the shale, the drill bit must be turned to run horizontally.

The technique of horizontal drilling was actually first applied to dentistry. In 1891, John Smalley Campbell (US Patent Number 459,152) described the idea that flexible shafts could be used to rotate drilling bits for dental applications, but he didn't exclude the notion that his invention might someday be used for other purposes: "It is obvious that its use is not confined thereto, but that it may be applied to flexible driving-shafts or cables of any other description."[5] Although the first recorded horizontal oil well was drilled in 1929 in Texas, it wasn't until the early 1980s that the process was improved and applied with some success.[6]

Likewise, one of the first uses of hydraulic fracturing had nothing to do with extracting oil or gas. Instead, Thomas Leonard Watson used an early form of this process in 1908 to separate granite from bedrock in order to study granites.[7] Hydraulic fracturing—using low volumes of water, not the high volumes used today—was introduced in the 1940s and was originally used to stimulate the flow of gas, and subsequently oil, from vertical wells.[8] In this way, the driller could extract oil or gas from relatively nonporous rock, such as shales, rather than simply from pockets of free oil or gas.

By the 1990s, the technology for modern-day horizontal drilling was married to fracturing with very high volumes of chemically laced water[9] (*slickwater*)—thus the term *horizontal drilling with high-volume hydraulic fracturing*—allowing operators to drill down and turn the bit horizontally within the layer of shale containing the fossil fuels, continuing the drilling for up to two miles.[10] The entire length of the well could then be hydraulically fractured, producing far more oil or gas. The idea was that large regions of the country (*shale plays*) sit on rocks containing fossil fuels that could be extracted with this process. By dividing these shale plays into spacing units of perhaps one square mile, the entire region could be drilled and enormous quantities of oil or gas could be extracted.

In 2008, Terry Engelder of Pennsylvania State University and Gary Lash of State University of New York at Fredonia calculated that the vast Marcellus and Utica Shales underlying parts of Ohio, West Virginia, Pennsylvania, New York, and Maryland contained almost 500 trillion cubic feet of gas.[11] They proposed that this vast reservoir of gas could be the nation's answer to energy independence, a flagging economy, high unemployment, and global warming. Along with other shale plays in Texas, Oklahoma, Colorado, Wyoming, Arkansas, North Dakota, and elsewhere in the United States, the nation would become the next Saudi Arabia of fossil fuels. Although we have little infrastructure to use methane as a fuel in transportation, and although multinational companies with no allegiance to our country are often the ones extracting our fossil fuels, the unconventional oil and gas revolution was also touted as a way of weaning ourselves off foreign oil.

But the more we learned about unconventional fossil fuel extraction, the more we realized that the prospects may not be as rosy as have been projected by the oil and gas industry. The US Geologic Survey reduced the original estimates of gas in the Marcellus region from 500 to 84 trillion cubic feet.[12] The lower estimate represents little more than three times the US yearly domestic gas use, with all of New York potentially contributing, at best, a six-month supply from the Marcellus Shale (not taking into account the plans for export of natural gas by multinational companies).[13] At least for New York, this is likely to be an overestimate, since only wells drilled in counties near the Pennsylvania border are likely be profitable.[14] Also, the output from shale gas wells has been found to decrease dramatically after the first year, suggesting that the production estimates may decrease further.[15] Moreover, when the price of natural gas was low in late 2013, the industry and the US government were prompted to search for more ways of using the product and converting terminals previously used to import gas into export terminals to send the gas to foreign markets. Whether any of the claims associated with the current "oil and gas boom" will stand up to careful scrutiny is a matter of ongoing debate, but large-scale industrial drilling has definitely moved into more densely populated areas and has garnered a massive amount of attention.

While the still-to-be-demonstrated economic benefits of unconventional fossil fuel extraction are continually promoted in the media and by the government, the environmental aspects have been given little or no attention until recently. With the growing awareness of the environmental impact of hydraulic fracturing, legions of grassroots organizers and environmental groups worldwide, who fear devastation of rural and urban landscapes, are now locked in a titanic struggle with large multinational corporations seeking to extract fossil fuels with unconventional techniques. While the overwhelming majority of the opposition to drilling has been peaceful, gas wells drilled in the sour-gas fields of Alberta, Canada, in the 1990s were met with some public resistance. There, grassroots activism apparently gave way to sabotage and violence.[16] Recent protests against shale gas exploration near an aboriginal reserve in the Canadian province of New Brunswick also turned violent.[17]

At least part of the reason for the forceful public reaction was the perceived danger of the process. *Sour gas* is a euphemism for a gas laced with highly toxic hydrogen sulfide, which may be released during the actual drilling of the well, as fugitive emissions from equipment, during incomplete combustion of flared gas, or when gas is vented. The flaring or venting is done before a pipeline is connected to the well and before production begins. It is important to note that gas emitted from oil wells being hydraulically fractured in North Dakota's Bakken Formation are left to flare or vent for long periods, sometimes years, because it is more expensive to capture the gas, process it, and move it along a pipeline than it is to burn it or release it into the atmosphere. The effects of drilling and flaring have been reported in environmental health studies.[18] And although stillbirths and other reproductive problems in cattle in these areas have been documented in the scientific literature, and reports of stillborn human infants have also surfaced, they have not been thoroughly investigated.

The problems do not stop with air pollution but also include water and soil pollution. Industry representatives often assert that millions of wells have been hydraulically fractured with not one instance of proven drinking-water contamination.[19] In response to the finding that between 2008 and 2013, the water supply of 161 homes in Pennsylvania was damaged by oil and gas drilling, we are told by the Pennsylvania Department of Environmental Protection (PADEP) that the industry will require an "adjustment period" to refine practices.[20] Also, Terry Engelder recently noted that the more hydraulic fracturing is used, the better the industry will get and that the current problems are necessary sacrifices during the period when the industry learns to do things more safely.[21] Thus, we are left with a bit of cognitive dissonance: the practice is perfectly safe and has been for sixty years, yet the industry needs time to get it right and we need to sacrifice while it perfects its methods.

When citing the lack of environmental contamination, the industry generally refers only to the hydraulic fracturing process itself—a small part of the entire life cycle of a gas or an oil well—and the industry does not state what level of proof of harm is acceptable. Because the shale is typically between 1,000 and 7,000 feet below the aquifer level, the drill bit must pass through the aquifer. This first step—that of punching a hole through a community's unprotected water supply, of disturbing the aquifer repeatedly with each well that is spudded (i.e., first drilled)—is seldom mentioned by the industry as a possible cause of the water quality and quantity changes observed in intensively drilled areas. Too often, we have spoken with families living in areas being actively drilled and whose water turned brown the same day each month, not unlike the schedule a driller might use to spud wells quickly on a multi-well pad.

After the vertical drilling, the well is cased in several layers of cement to protect the shallow layers, including aquifers. A large horizontal well requires approximately five million gallons of water laced with silica and other chemicals (approximately 0.5 to 2 percent of the total fluid). These chemicals range from the relatively benign to the highly toxic. The fluid is injected into the well at high pressure to fracture the shale. If the cement casing is done properly, the fluid may not be able to reach the aquifer during the fracturing process. In the cases where aquifers have been contaminated because of a faulty cement casing, it is not counted as contamination by hydraulic fracturing by industry representatives but simply a case of an imperfection in the cement. This is of little comfort to families whose well water has been compromised to such an extent that complete filtration systems must be installed, or "water buffalos"—holding approximately two thousand gallons of water—must be provided. Following hydraulic fracturing, the pressure is released and wastewater, oil, gas, or a mixture of these returns to the surface, presenting another opportunity to contaminate aquifers if the cement job is faulty. Within the first fifteen years following the drilling of a well, data from the US Mineral Management Service suggest that up to 50 percent of well casings do not adequately control the migration of hydrocarbons ("sustained casing pressure") in offshore wells.[22] Although the proliferation of unconventional wells is a relatively recent phenomenon, Pennsylvania data indicate that the track record onshore thus far follows the same trend as the offshore wells.[23] Also, channels forming outside the cement casing have been known to allow at least methane into drinking-water aquifers.[24]

The initial wastewater, referred to as *flowback*, contains a portion of the hydraulic fracturing fluid; later, substances trapped for hundreds of millions of years in the shale layers flow to the surface along with the gas or oil as "produced water." Thus, wastewater can be as toxic as, or more toxic than, hydraulic fracturing fluid, as witnessed by farmers whose herds' reproductive capacity was greatly diminished after the cattle were exposed to leaky impoundments. Other witnesses include pet owners whose dogs died soon after playing in puddles of waste fluids spread on the road or after lapping fluid from unfenced impoundments. The problem is that the well operator must now deal with millions of gallons of toxic fluid in the form of wastewater that has been left in pits to evaporate, recycled to be used in other wells (increasing the concentration of toxic chemicals), spread on our roads as deicing fluid or to suppress dust, given to wastewater-treatment plants that are ill equipped to handle these toxicants, or returned to the earth by injection into deep wells (sometimes resulting in small earthquakes as we learned from a family surrounded by injection wells in central Arkansas). Each of these dubious solutions to the wastewater issue has been associated with environmental and health problems.

But certainly, you would think that citizens would be protected from environmental and health impacts through the strict enforcement of the Safe Drinking Water Act (SDWA) by the US Environmental Protection Agency (EPA). The EPA had for many years considered hydraulic fracturing outside its regulatory authority. However, a class action lawsuit brought by the Legal Environmental Assistance Foundation (LEAF) in 1994 challenged the EPA's stance. The suit concerned hydraulic fracturing in coal bed methane wells in the Black Warrior Basin of Alabama.[25] The Eleventh Circuit US Court of Appeals ruled in favor of LEAF in 1997 and required the EPA to regulate the process. In 1999, the EPA began a study of the risks that hydraulic fracturing in coal-bed methane reservoirs posed to drinking water. However, during the four years of the study, the Bush administration came into office, with the former CEO of Halliburton, Richard Cheney, serving as vice president. Cheney's energy task force repeatedly touted the benefits of hydraulic fracturing, and in 2004, the EPA study was released, concluding that hydraulic fracturing posed no serious threat to drinking water in coal-bed methane reservoirs. Soon after the release of the study, an EPA scientist, Weston Wilson, wrote a letter to Congress outlining the conflicts of interests in the panel that reviewed the data and the political pressure to produce the conclusion favored by the vice president. Wilson's assertions aside, in 2005, the SDWA definition of underground injection was specified by Congress to exclude hydraulic fracturing. This act of Congress, known as the "Halliburton Loophole," has removed the EPA from any regulation of hydraulic fracturing, leaving regulation up to the individual states.

One might also consider the danger posed by the millions of gallons of hydraulic fracturing fluid and the toxic flowback fluid at the surface as an important regulatory issue for the EPA. Here again, the EPA has little authority, as the agency regulation states: "Drilling fluids, produced waters, and other wastes associated with the exploration, development, or production of . . . natural gas [are considered] . . . solid wastes which are not hazardous wastes."[26] That is, no matter how toxic the liquid, if it is produced in the exploration, development, or production of gas, it is by definition nontoxic. Defining a substance as nontoxic in this manner is similar to a vegetarian's defining a rare, juicy steak as a vegetable and eating it with gusto.

The EPA has recently undertaken a study of hydraulic fracturing and its impact on drinking-water resources and may revise some of these apparently outdated regulations.[27] Despite this ongoing study, the Office of the Inspector General of the EPA issued a report acknowledging the limited air-emissions data for oil and gas production: "With limited data, human health risks are uncertain, states may design incorrect or ineffective emission control strategies, and EPA's decisions about regulating industry may be misinformed."[28] Currently, regulations are set by the individual states, and the extent of regulation and degree of enforcement vary widely among the states that allow high-volume hydraulic fracturing. According to Lisa Jackson, the former administrator of the EPA, "The scale has really gone up astronomically: a thousand wells a year in the Fort Worth area. Remember, oil and gas drilling and development is primarily in this country regulated at the state level. States like Texas, states like Wyoming, states like Pennsylvania, are going to have to step up. We do have cases where we do believe we see many cases of groundwater contamination and drinking-water contamination that are if not brought on entirely by natural gas production, were exacerbated by it. Not just methane, which is natural gas, but other contaminants as well."[29]

The question that we are left with is, do the costs outweigh the benefits? That is, to what extent can we tolerate the inevitable environmental degradation that accompanies extraction of hydrocarbons via high-volume hydraulic fracturing? Can we bring renewable sources of energy online rapidly so that the extraction of fossil fuels by any means is less attractive? There are no easy answers to these questions. We can marvel at the accomplishments of geologists and engineers who have devised methods for extracting these natural resources. But the major questions that remain are not in the realm of the engineer. The questions are now of a biological, environmental, and medical nature. Simply put, we are not certain of the public health implications of large-scale industrial oil and gas drilling.

Public health information is difficult to obtain. Reproductive problems and cancer may take years to develop, and in our mobile society, proving a causal relationship between an environmental risk factor and a particular disease can be difficult or impossible. Some environmentalists often invoke the "precautionary principle," which states that if an action is suspected of causing harm, then the burden of proof is on the entity taking such action. In the case of the fossil fuel industry, the precautionary principle would suggest that this industry has the obligation to prove that its actions do not cause public harm. The fossil fuel industry, however, seems to have taken a page from the tobacco industry playbook. That is, if a link between drilling operations and public health cannot be proven definitively, then the link is rejected, effectively putting the burden of proof on the victim.

Cass Sunstein, a renowned legal scholar from the University of Chicago, argues that the precautionary principle is inherently incoherent in the sense that risks exist both by taking and avoiding a particular action.[30] However, if we move away from the strict interpretation of the precautionary principle, we can begin to define the risks involved in large-scale gas and oil drilling and to assign the burden of proof for avoiding a certain level of harm. This will require careful scientific studies of the health effects of drilling operations. But how can we obtain useful information in a reasonable time? The answer, we believe, is to consider animals, children, and fossil fuel workers as sentinels of human health.

Using animals as sentinels has been championed by Peter Rabinowitz of Yale University,[31] and we discussed this approach to studying health impacts of gas drilling operations in a recent paper.[32] We agree with the National Academy of Sciences Committee on Animals as Sentinels of Environmental Health Hazards, which noted, "The primary goal of an animal sentinel system is to identify harmful chemicals or chemical mixtures in the environment *before* they might otherwise be detected through human epidemiologic studies or toxicologic studies in laboratory animals. Once identified, exposures could be minimized until methods can be devised to determine specific etiologic agents. Animal sentinel systems themselves are not the answer to the latter problem but might provide additional valuable time in which to search for the answer."[33]

In addition to animals, children are inadvertent sentinels. Because of their higher metabolic rates and immature neurologic and detoxifying systems, children are at higher risk of developing adverse health effects from environmental hazards, including those from nearby industrial operations. As we update our study, we are finding more cases where children are often the first in the family to become ill. Initial results on babies living near industrial gas operations in Pennsylvania have demonstrated an increased prevalence of low birth weight and a reduction of five-minute APGAR scores (assessment of appearance, pulse, grimace, activity, and respiration at birth),[34] indicating that infants born in intensively drilled areas may suffer health impacts starting at birth. But oil and gas workers—with the highest likelihood of direct exposures to chemicals and the highest mortality rates of any industry—are perhaps our best, yet least studied, sentinels.[35]

As we studied the impacts of unconventional drilling, we spoke with families about their health and the health of their pets and farm animals. All the families we interviewed live near industrial fossil fuel operations in one of the major shale plays in the United States, including Pennsylvania, Ohio, Texas, Louisiana, Colorado, North Dakota, Arkansas, and New York. Former employees of the fossil fuel industry and concerned citizens throughout the country referred us to people whose water and air had become severely affected, whose animals were dying, and whose lives were being turned upside down by the oil and gas industry. While each story, each context, each timeline of events was different, we were alarmed by what we kept hearing over and over again from people in very different situations hundreds of miles apart:

> "Water dispensers and water buffaloes have replaced our
>   water sources."
> "All of my puppies were born dead."
> "I have no calves this year."
> "My vet can't figure out what's happening to my animals."
> "We had to leave our home to escape the bad air."
> "I had no choice but to leave my goats and pigs behind."
> "I leased to keep my land, but I lost my farm."
> "We all have headaches, nosebleeds, and rashes."
> "I'd move out, but I can't afford it."
> "We are not living; we are merely existing."

We decided that these stories needed to be told. Almost everyone with whom we have spoken is either involved in litigation against the fossil fuel industry or seriously contemplating it. Some people distrust and fear this industry, while others remain staunch supporters despite the devastating consequences of drilling in their own lives. Some people are former oil and gas industry employees, while, for others, the experiences they described were their first contact with oil and gas drilling.

We have divided this book into three sections. The first section, chapters 1 through 4, chronicles the lives of families and their pets—

dogs, cats, horses, goats, rabbits, pigs, chickens, and a donkey. Because companion animals live among us, sometimes never leaving our sides, changes in their behavior and health are quickly and easily observed. As such, the companion animals in these stories served as bellwethers, giving their owners early warning that something was amiss.

The second section—chapters 5 through 7—encompasses farmers and food-producing animals, largely beef cattle. Although the farmers described in this section professed fondness for their animals, a crucial issue was the economic effects of the deaths of their animals and the loss of reproductive capacity. An associated problem is the potential introduction of toxicants into the food supply directly from crops or exposed animals (from meat, milk, eggs, or cheese) or indirectly through rendering, where animals' flesh and bones are turned into products used to feed other animals or, in some cases, humans (through the production of lard from animal fat). This illustrates the important point that the effects of industrialized gas drilling have the potential to affect people in areas far from active drilling regions.

In the last section (chapters 8 and 9), we depict the issues surrounding unconventional gas drilling and environmental justice. We illustrate how one family living in a disenfranchised, poor community surrounded by shale gas operations not only copes with the loss of clean water and fresh air, but also survives as a unit by sacrificing for each other.

Each of the stories is told in the first person from the perspective of one of us (Michelle Bamberger), who conducted most of the interviews. For each story told here, there are many more families that could tell similar tales. We think of the travails of the people and animals in our stories as illustrations of the impacts we all face from industrialized gas drilling.

When we first began speaking with people, we simply asked, What happened to you and what happened to your animals? After the first few interviews, it became obvious that to tell a complete story, we needed the details of drilling: we asked about seismic testing; about the distance of the well pad to water sources; the name of the drilling company; when the well was drilled and fractured; about the distance of the wastewater impoundment to the water well and to springs, creeks, and ponds; about trucks spreading and dumping wastewater; about pipeline rup-

tures and when the well was flared; about compressor stations and processing plants in the neighborhood; about the location of deep-injection
wells; and about the occurrence of earthquakes. We asked about all of
this, in addition to the results of water, air, and soil tests, veterinary and
human health records, and permission to contact veterinarians.

People provided as much information as they had available to them.
Not everyone had a regular veterinarian. Cattle farmers, especially beef
cattle farmers, often cover their own routine veterinary care. Not everyone had predrilling tests done, and those who did most often consented
to driller initiated tests that were often incomplete, lacking results for
volatile and semivolatile organic and radioactive compounds. Tests are
expensive: only one person we spoke with ran complete water and air
tests through a private laboratory before and after drilling began, spending more than $4,000 in one year. Veterinary testing, including screen-
ing for toxicants, was not done routinely, especially in large animals, for
the same reason. We found that well-documented cattle cases were the
anomaly: necropsies (animal autopsies) were usually not done, screening
for toxicants was even rarer, and the names of all chemicals used in drilling and fracturing operations were not known. Without basic testing
and knowledge of all the chemicals used, definitive proof linking oil and
gas drilling operations to animal or human health problems is difficult
to obtain.

We quickly learned that people were experiencing the same problems with conventional wells (shallow or deep vertical drilling with low-
volume hydraulic fracturing) as they were with unconventional wells
(horizontal drilling with high-volume hydraulic fracturing). But because
of the scale of industrialized oil and gas operations occurring throughout the country, unconventional wells were more commonly associated
with animal and human health problems.

Perhaps the most consistent finding from case to case and one that
most people discussed at length was the irresponsible behavior of the
drilling companies and the state environmental regulatory agencies in
handling problems occurring after the onset of oil or gas drilling. In
most cases, people complained bitterly of unfair treatment during the
process of reporting, testing, and remediation of a contamination incident. Several people also complained of occasions where friends were

harassed and intimidated at work when they spoke out. In several instances, documentation of cases was thwarted due to the signing of a nondisclosure agreement.

Nondisclosure agreements often make the information on contamination incidents and health effects impossible to obtain, as we found while investigating several cases. These agreements are signed in exchange for compensation in the form of cash, an offer to pay for all settlement expenses, an offer to buy the owner's property, and payment for medical expenses of the owners and, rarely, their animals. After the agreement is signed, further comment is prohibited. If the owner breaks the nondisclosure agreement (the confidentiality is breached), the oil or gas company can then hold back on cash or other payments, and the owner then may be liable for damages. Nondisclosure agreements are common in all areas of business and are often essential to protect intellectual property, but when used to block documentation of health problems associated with oil or gas drilling (or any other public health issue), these agreements are clearly a misuse of this important business tool.

From a veterinary medicine standpoint, two issues arose during these interviews that disturbed and unsettled us. The first concerned food safety and economics. All of the farmers we interviewed found themselves financially squeezed by gas drilling. In many cases, farmers experienced heavy losses due to death and reproductive failure of their herds in association with drilling-related events; in one case, losses were compounded by long quarantine hold times of the herd following wastewater exposure. A number of farmers spent thousands of dollars on environmental testing. As a result, many of them felt pressed to send their exposed food-producing animals to slaughter. In all except one case, exposed animals that didn't survive or couldn't walk went directly to the renderer. To our knowledge, none of these animals were tested before slaughter or rendering, and farms in areas testing positive for air, soil, and water contamination are still producing meat, eggs, and dairy products for human consumption without testing the animals or the products. This situation makes it likely that some of these chemicals could appear in food products made from these animals. On the economics side, farmers not only lost animals but also lost pastureland and hayfields, depending on the placement of the access road, well pad, wastewater and freshwater impoundments, drilling muds pit, compressor station, and pipeline. Most of the farmers and other people we spoke with received no compensation from the driller for the loss of their animals, the loss of their land, or for the treatment of the animal and human health problems they encountered since oil or gas drilling came to their neighborhoods.

The second issue emerged during interviews with veterinarians. We were not surprised to hear that many veterinarians were seeing similar cases of health related issues associated with oil or gas drilling. We did not expect, however, to hear that fear of loss of clients was driving some veterinarians to avoid speaking out and more thoroughly investigating suspect cases by sending them on to necropsy. One large-animal veterinarian requested permission to submit cases under another veterinarian's account, to avoid being associated with the results, and the possible loss of business.

At the outset, we did not intend to collect specific information on human health issues associated with oil and gas drilling exposures. However, as many owners reported similar symptoms in themselves and their pets or livestock, it soon became obvious that both people and animals were being affected by the same set of circumstances. We decided early on that it was crucial to ask specifics on human health: how it was affected, and to what degree. We also found that the human health data were another important piece of the timeline we generated for each case. For example, we charted the dates when drilling and hydraulic fracturing occurred; when water, air, and soil quality changed; and when animals and their owners fell ill. Our stories tell of how people were affected in the short term, and now, as we continue to collect updates on these interviews, we are able to describe the long-term effects in owners as well as their animals. After more than two years of following our cases, we have observed that health impacts significantly decreased over time for families and animals moving away from intensively drilled areas, or living in areas where the level of industrial activity has decreased; otherwise, health impacts have remained the same. We have also observed that in food animals, both respiratory problems and growth problems (stunting and failure to thrive) have increased over time. This is interesting, especially in light of the epidemiological studies of human births occurring in intensively drilled areas (mentioned above).

In the process of reviewing medical records on animal owners, we were surprised and dismayed to learn that several physicians failed to record their patients' history of exposure to oil or gas drilling operations on the medical records, despite the patient's oral history at the time of the office appointment. We can only hope that as awareness of health issues linked to unconventional oil and gas drilling increases in the medical community, all physicians will include such history on intake and will report such cases to their respective state health departments.

As discussed previously, in comparing the health effects of drilling-related activities on animals to those of their owners, it is not surprising that both small and large animals should experience more health problems sooner and to a greater degree than their owners because in most situations, they are exposed to the environment for longer periods than their owners. They don't drive to work or run errands: they are subjected to the air, soil, and water provided to them, however good or bad it may be. This difference emerged in the interviews, in sometimes unexpected and astonishing ways.

When we began speaking with people, we couldn't have imagined the void we were filling by taking this project on. The updates never end, because in many cases exposures never end: contamination of water, air, and soil is difficult if not impossible to remedy. Because known carcinogens, mutagens, and endocrine disruptors are used in industrial gas drilling operations, and because these chemicals can cause long-term health problems to many systems in the body at very low concentrations (parts per billion or less), we expect to be following the health issues of animals and their owners for many more years.

After countless hours of listening and recording these stories, we realized that our role was not only one of interviewer, but also of crisis counselor. People tell us stories they can tell no one else. They need to talk. They are like victims of a rape. The rapist says, "Be quiet or I will kill you." In some of the stories we have documented, the drilling companies have told the people, "No more water." These people plead and beg for water. They live on the edge of sanity, day to day, trying to get by, but how can you live without water? Some people are afraid that their water buffalos will be taken away—if they were lucky enough to have received one when their water became undrinkable—so they say, "No, I can't speak out. No, you can't use my name," and then they tell us their stories. Some whisper, some shout. We feel their sense of relief on getting their stories out, like getting rid of the rot inside, making you sick. We invite them to let it out, dump it on us, the people listening, trying to find out something, anything, as much as possible about what awaits should their fate become our fate.

ONE

FAMILIES AND THEIR PETS

A farm close to a small town would seem to be an ideal place to raise a family, with fresh air, clean water, open space, animals both domestic and wild, and only the sounds of children playing. But despite our idyllic view of the countryside, the jobs have largely moved overseas, and in many areas of the country, people are struggling to make ends meet, raise a family, and take care of beloved animals. In shale gas country, this is also where the riches lay, deep underground. In Pennsylvania, some people embrace the shale gas revolution, hoping for a better life. Others accept it, hoping for the best and praying that it will work out for them. And still others are deeply skeptical. In chapters 2, 3, and 4, we illustrate how very different families in different parts of Pennsylvania face the challenge of living amid shale gas drilling and find unique ways of dealing with trouble.

As much as parents or animal owners would like to think of themselves as protectors of their child or pet, it is ironic that both children and animals are actually more like the canaries in the coal mine. Because children are smaller than adults and tend to eat, drink and breathe more air relative to their body weights, they tend to be more affected by environmental insults. Add to this an increased sensitivity of the still-forming nervous system and a reduced ability to detoxify substances,[1] and we can state with some assurance that children are particularly susceptible to chemicals in the environment. While children are sentinels, for many reasons animals are even more so. When families leave for work and school, their animals are often left at home either in the house, barn, or yard, increasing exposure times. Whereas children can be given bottled water to drink, few people can afford to buy bottled water for a horse. So for different reasons, we think of both children and pet or farm animals as sentinels of environmental disease. They are the first to fall sick, and the symptoms and consequences can be dire.

Picture for a moment a quiet country lane barely wide enough for two cars to pass, with some homes and farms that have been in the family for generations. With dark skies at night and clean air and water, this is the perfect place for a family to live, to care for a dog and maybe a horse and a few chickens. On the other hand, while the good things in life are present in abundance, it may not be the most prosperous area of the country. In many cases, the land has been leased to drilling companies for many years with little or no impact. The leases were for a dollar or two an acre and if a small gas well was drilled, few people other than the landowner ever heard about it. It is in this context that landsmen appeared on the scene, offering more lucrative leases, with little indication that life was about to change for people living in such communities. Many people signed leases hoping for a better life, while others signed thinking that with a lease, they could have more control over what was about to happen.

In many, if not most, cases, people welcomed this newfound potential for wealth. One individual who had worked for many years for an oil and gas company was thrilled by the prospect of leasing his farm. He had known gas wells as a company insider and thought that his dream of having a working farm in a beautiful area of southwestern Pennsylvania could easily coexist with the small changes brought about by a well or two on his property. What he didn't know was that the lease he had signed allowed the company to place multiple large drilling pads on his farm, each pad with several horizontal wells. As it turns out, the dream of a working farm never materialized. He did build a pond and stocked it with fish, more for the pleasure of fishing and enjoying nature. The next step was to purchase some cows and start a beef cattle herd. He thought that it would be easy—he could just negotiate where the access roads would go and where the drilling pads would be located. Instead, the drilling pad was placed just above his fishpond, and the access road ran past his children's bedrooms. After his fishpond was contaminated by runoff from the well pad and he caught workers on his property stealing his machinery, he realized that his dream was slowly turning into a train wreck. But he was one of the lucky ones. He and his family escaped with their health mostly intact, and we heard his story while he was living at his mother's home, the farm a distant and painful memory.

But was this an isolated instance? Could all of the woes that we heard from him be exaggerations? To look into this further, we visited a neighbor who keeps goats and fish as pets and had lived in the same house for forty years, a rented property with the mineral rights leased to the drilling company. Around the time that the would-be farmer's fish-pond was allegedly contaminated, the neighbor found that his goats were experiencing severe neurological symptoms, and five of eight suddenly died. At about the same time, he had replaced the water in a small pond where he kept koi with his well water. To his amazement, all of the fish died soon after. He removed the water and restocked the pond with water from a remote source and has had healthy fish to this day. While dealing with the tragedies associated with their pets, both the neighbor and his elderly mother began experiencing rashes and a distinct change in the smell and color of their well water.

Can we prove that drilling on the farm specifically caused these health issues? Neither water nor air testing was done prior to drilling, and only water testing was done afterward. Given the forty-year history in the same home and multiple instances of human and animal sickness associated temporally with drilling and hydraulically fracturing multiple wells, at least the suspicion is raised that the problem may have arisen from recent unconventional drilling operations. We will never know the answer for sure, but the question that we raise is where the burden of proof lies.

Around the corner from these two neighbors, a family with two small children was living in their newly built dream house. The land that they purchased to build their home was part of a parcel that had been subdivided by the previous owner. The mineral rights for the land upon which they built their house had been leased, and on the adjacent property, both the mineral rights and the surface rights had been leased. Soon after the house was completed, drilling activity commenced in earnest. Four gas wells were drilled on the adjacent property, along with a compressor station and a wastewater impoundment; also nearby were buried pipelines and a gas processing plant.

The family began to experience burning eyes and sore throats, part of a constellation of symptoms that we refer to as *shale gas syndrome*, which also includes headaches, nosebleeds, vomiting, diarrhea, and skin rashes. These symptoms, of course, can be caused by a variety of things but are typical of people we spoke to living near shale gas operations. Predrilling testing of water was not done because this family's water well was drilled after shale gas operations had begun; likewise, no predrilling air testing was done. After family members began to feel sick, some water testing was done both by the family and the drilling company, with conflicting results. In an effort to protect the children, the family settled with the gas company. Initially, the courts sealed all information about this case with a nondisclosure agreement, effectively removing the evidence of harm from public and scientific scrutiny.

In hopes of obtaining the family's health records, we joined several other individuals and organizations to file an amicus brief in a case to have the evidence unsealed. The case was eventually unsealed,[2] revealing a settlement of $750,000 and affidavits the family was compelled to sign as a part of the settlement. The affidavits stated that no medical evidence definitively connects the children's health problems to gas operations and that the children were in good health.[3] In fact, the children were prohibited from speaking in public about the oil and gas industry for the remainder of their lives, a potential violation of First Amendment rights.[4]

Before a judge unsealed this case after extended litigation, we had some idea of the facts of the case but could not study the evidence further, because the nondisclosure agreement effectively bought silence in the public domain. The reversal of a nondisclosure agreement is extremely rare. Let us imagine if other industries that have the potential to affect public health could use the simple tool of a nondisclosure agreement. What if a drug company were to bring a drug to market and when the drug began widespread use, a measurable fraction of the population taking the drug died of heart attacks? It might be difficult to know for certain if the drug was the cause of the fatal heart attacks without further study. Perhaps the simple solution for the drug company would be to pay the families of the victims to keep silent and have all prescription records sealed by court order. The company could then continue to sell the product and make large profits, with the occasional collateral damage. The action would avoid the messy business of an investigation and further study. Of course, this could never be tolerated and a full investigation with complete disclosure of the facts would be required.

Getting back to the fresh air, clean water, and quiet surroundings—the reasons all of the families gave us for living in the countryside—we can only imagine their surprise when the first earthmoving equipment arrived and the drill pad and wastewater impoundment were readied for action. This was a larger operation than anyone had expected. The West (Colorado, Wyoming, Oklahoma, and Texas) had seen these large wells—as we discovered while documenting several cases in Colorado—but they were generally off the radar of anyone living in the Midwest or Eastern states. An individual living outside Pittsburgh described it this way: "We have been invaded." It is important to think about the significance of this statement. This is not someone living in a quiet village in New England; this is someone living in the middle of a mining area, where coal and coal-bed methane are routinely extracted from the ground, with significant environmental impact.

The initial invasion takes the form of trucks, many trucks. First the large earthmoving equipment arrives to re-sculpt the land and create the drilling pad and impoundments to hold wastewater and drilling fluids, muds, and cuttings (solid material that the drill bit produces as it advances through the rock). Then the drilling rig is moved in, followed within a few weeks by an endless stream of trucks carrying water, sand, and toxic chemicals for the hydraulic fracturing. On quiet country roads that sometimes are only ten or twenty feet from a home—roads that never see more than a handful of cars and trucks over the course of the day—truck after truck idles, sometimes speeding by, but always spewing out diesel fumes laced with benzene. Benzene is a potent carcinogen and not what most parents would like their children to breathe or what most dog owners consider healthy for their canine companions. This is the norm—what happens when things proceed as planned.

While the industry and some state regulatory agencies insist that problems are nonexistent or at least manageable, the drilling and hydraulic fracturing processes can pose risks to water and air. The drilling process itself often contacts aquifers, in some cases aquifers that supply drinking water to families in the vicinity of the well. The well is then separated from drinking water by several layers of concrete, but this concrete has been known to fail. In at least one case, most of the wells in a particular area in northeast Pennsylvania required repairs because of a faulty casing in each well. The well is drilled down and the bit is turned to run horizontally into the shale formation of interest. For the Marcellus or Utica Shales in Pennsylvania, the shale formation is thousands of feet below the drinking-water aquifers. This fact has been used to argue in favor of the safety of the process. However, according to industry estimates, fractures can extend vertically up to two thousand feet.[5] In areas where the formation is shallow (e.g., the Marcellus Shale in parts of New York State), direct interaction with aquifers could be a problem. Also, connections with natural faults and abandoned gas wells (tens of thousands of unknown and abandoned wells exist in New York[6] and Pennsylvania) can bring fluids from the fracturing process into contact with an aquifer.

In addition to potential aquifer contamination, surface spills of both hydraulic fracturing fluids and the toxic and radioactive substances brought up with the gas have been documented and have contaminated ponds and streams. The wastewater brought up from the wells during the production phase contains high levels of salt. After all, these shale formations are nothing more than ancient oceans where the seawater has dried, leaving the salt behind. This wastewater can be spread on roads in New York and Pennsylvania to control dust and to melt ice and snow. But it is not only salt (sodium chloride) that is spread on the roads. The wastewater also contains organic compounds, heavy metals, and radioactive materials, the composition of which changes with time even after the well is put into production. Only minimal testing is required to sell this waste for spreading on roads, and we have witnessed illegal spreading for which there are no controls. This becomes a problem because of leakage into surface water, farmland, and even homeowner's yards. When the wastewater dries on a dirt road, the substances become part of the dust that people breathe while walking, biking, or driving on the road.

It is no surprise that health issues have been noted, given all of the potential problems associated with normal operations, accidental spills, and air and water contamination. During a presentation at the College of Physicians in Philadelphia, Raina Rippel, the director of the Southwest Pennsylvania Environmental Health Project (www.environmental healthproject.org), a clinic near Pittsburgh that sees affected individuals every day, said, choking back tears, "You have to believe that these things are happening . . . These are people who have lived on this land for generations . . . Their quality of life has been destroyed . . . The debate over whether there are health impacts needs to end: there *are* health impacts." The problem we face is that the symptoms of shale gas syndrome, while fairly consistent among those that have been heavily exposed to shale gas extraction, are not unique. Headache, GI upset, nosebleeds, rash, and burning of the eyes, nose, and throat have multiple causes, and proving without a doubt that the symptoms are caused by proximity to gas and oil wells is difficult at best. We see consistency of symptoms, we can show that the symptoms started when the drilling started, we can show that the symptoms go away when the people or animals leave the area, but this is not scientific proof; this is a correlation.

So how do we obtain proof? The typical approach in environmental toxicology is to show that a toxic substance exists in the environment, then show the pathway that the substance enters the body, and finally correlate the symptoms with exposure to the toxic chemical. In a case associated with gas distribution, Erin Brockovich and Edward Masry settled a lawsuit in 1996 demonstrating that hexavalent chromium, a known carcinogen used to fight corrosion in the cooling tower of the Hinkley Compressor Station near San Francisco, leaked into wastewater that was put into unlined ponds near the station. The hexavalent chromium subsequently contaminated groundwater in the area, allegedly affecting the health of nearby residents. Relative to understanding the effects of shale gas extraction on public and animal health, the Brockovich case was comparatively simple in that a single substance was involved. This is not to understate the complexity of the hexavalent chromium case, but rather to emphasize the difficulty of studying shale gas syndrome. We are dealing with multiple chemicals of varying toxicity, some of which are known and some unknown, with multiple, often concomitant exposure pathways, and insufficient pre- and postdrilling testing of air, water, soil, people, and animals.

From our case studies, we know that animals and humans have symptoms that correlate in time with gas and oil drilling operations, particularly unconventional wells. We know that health clinics in Pennsylvania and Colorado report that people living near shale gas operations have symptoms similar to what we have seen in people and are now calling shale gas syndrome. We know that water wells in areas near shale gas operations have been contaminated by methane that has the isotopic signature of shale gas.[7] That is, using tests that determine the isotopes of carbon and hydrogen in the methane gas, scientists can determine if the gas is produced by organisms near the surface (biogenic methane) or if it comes from the shale layers deep within the earth (thermogenic methane). This is important because many water wells throughout Pennsylvania and New York are contaminated by low levels of biogenic methane that are unrelated to gas drilling. But we rarely have the smoking gun: this compound came from the gas well, ended up in the drinking water, was consumed by these people or these animals, and has caused this sickness. We have correlations, low levels of a multitude of chemicals, and little information on the effects of these chemicals and, particularly, the effects of combinations of chemicals on humans and animals. The data are lacking, and the statistical odds are against us.

If 2-butoxyethanol shows up in a homeowner's drinking-water well, do we assume that it is because the resident was using Windex to clean her windows, or can we admit the possibility that it came from the ten shale gas wells within a mile of her home? When a well is drilled and hydraulically fractured, and residents near the gas well see persistent and marked changes in the color, smell, and taste of their water unlike anything they have seen before, do we simply dismiss this as normal variation in water quality? A representative for a large gas company once told us that he is tired of hearing about changes in the color and taste of the water from residents near their gas wells, and the only thing that matters is chemical analysis. While no one can dispute that chemical analysis is the ideal, the statement comes fraught with multiple complicated issues that have not been adequately resolved.

Simply put, the issues are cost, ownership, choice of tests, secrecy, sensitivity, and interpretation. States have varying regulations, but testing of water wells in the area before drilling a gas well is becoming more common. However, testing results and the choice of tests belong to the party that pays for the test. This can be the homeowner, the drilling company, the state government, or the federal government (the US Environmental Protection Agency, EPA). Both states and drilling companies differ in what is tested and what is disclosed to the homeowner. According to court records, the Pennsylvania Department of Environmental Protection (PADEP) withheld complete test results of several toxic metals from a private water well located near a shale gas drilling site.[8] The homeowner is not given the list of substances to be used prior to drilling, so that testing must generally be limited to a subset of chemicals that may be used or may be present in the flowback water (the wastewater that returns to the surface within the first few weeks during and after hydraulic fracturing, and is composed mainly of hydraulic fracturing fluids).

Furthermore, testing is expensive (at least $500 per test), which can be prohibitive for a low-income individual living near a well but not part of the drilling unit and thus not anticipating royalties. As noted above, prior to drilling, the residents in the area are not routinely informed about the chemicals that will be used on the drilling site. Depending upon the state, this information may be revealed only to the regulatory agency. After the well has been drilled, an interested party can visit the FracFocus website (www.fracfocus.org) to obtain a partial list of the chemicals used in the drilling process. Because the information becomes available only after the well has been completed, the information is useless if a person wishes to conduct predrilling testing. Moreover, only chemicals that are not proprietary are reported, and any reporting is at the discretion of the drilling company. While this may be of some use in later tests, FracFocus does not provide the tools needed to design a comprehensive predrilling test.

Once the well is drilled and hydraulically fractured, if water quality changes, testing may be repeated. Again, ownership, disclosure of the results, and the prohibitive costs of the tests are at issue. But at this stage, we have to consider the sensitivity and interpretation of the tests. The maximum contaminant level, or MCL, is used to interpret whether a substance can cause adverse health effects in a public water system. MCLs are set by the EPA under the Safe Drinking Water Act (SDWA)[9]

and also by some state agencies. The SDWA has been enormously successful in improving public drinking water, but for the purposes of testing water wells in shale gas regions, there are some serious drawbacks.
MCLs are based on the idea that toxic substances have only one effect
(injury, disease, or death) at a particular threshold level and above. But it
is well known that many toxic substances can affect multiple physiologi-
cal processes and at different concentrations. In some cases, for example, certain endocrine disruptors, low concentrations can even be more
toxic than higher concentrations.[10] If we take a step further and consider the probability that multiple toxic substances can be present, the
use of the MCL as a standard for judging the quality of drinking water
degrades further. We know almost nothing about the health effects of
mixtures of toxic substances, and it is likely that the "safe" level of a
mixture cannot be judged by the individual MCLs.[11]

MCLs may not be available for substances found in well water for at
least two reasons. The first is simply that the EPA or a state agency has
not evaluated certain chemicals. Several people we interviewed are en-
rolled in the EPA's study of the potential impacts of hydraulic fracturing
on drinking-water resources, begun in 2010 and expected to continue at
least through 2014.[12] In this study, a wide range of constituents are
tested, but most lack primary MCLs. Drinking water may be deemed
safe for consumption despite the presence of such chemicals, because
there is no regulation stating that they are unsafe. In the Pennsylvania
case described above, the stated reason the PADEP withheld complete
water test results was that several metals were below the MCL or had no
MCL.[13] The other reason for the lack of an MCL is that routine tests
are not sensitive enough to measure low concentrations of a substance.
In this case, the EPA can mandate "Treatment Techniques,"[14] which are
procedures to remove such a contaminant if it were present in drinking
water. This is fine for public water-treatment plants, but is not applica-
ble to private well water. In the final analysis, we are left with MCLs that
have been useful for improving public drinking water, but have more
limited use in understanding water tests for private wells, particularly
those suspected of contamination by gas and oil drilling in the area.

Given the difficulties of predrilling testing and the interpretation of results, contamination of water is extremely difficult to prove, particularly for the homeowner of limited means. Proving that the presence of a chemical or, much more likely, a mixture of chemicals resulted in a particular symptom is even more difficult. But this is only one type of exposure. Air testing is more challenging and more expensive than water testing, and exposure levels are less well documented. Contamination by microbes is an area that is almost entirely unknown in this field. We know that even at the elevated pressures and extreme salt concentrations of the shale layers, bacteria and archaea (single-celled microorganisms with no nucleus or other membrane-bound organelles) are present and may be quite different from the organisms found at the surface.[15] Bactericides are used in hydraulic fracturing fluid to kill bacteria and avoid bacterial films that would impede the flow of gas to the surface. Making fracturing chemicals more "green" might have the unintended consequence of bringing viable, uncharacterized microbes to the surface.

We can do much better to protect public health with further research into the effects of chemicals used deep underground and those returning to the surface. In particular, we need to know more about long-term and low-dose effects as well as the effects of combinations of toxic substances. Finally, we need to understand the microbes that are brought back to the surface with the wastewater. Currently, these microorganisms can escape any detection in water tests and could present a significant health problem at low levels.

Given the difficulties in proving without a doubt that unconventional fossil fuel extraction has contaminated water and air and led to illness, it is perhaps easy to understand why we hear the constant refrain that this is a safe process that has been used for many years without problems. As is often said, absence of proof of harm cannot be equated to absence of harm, and we need to do more to protect the people living in shale gas country.

We illustrate the issues raised here with the stories of three families in different parts of Pennsylvania. They have all experienced health problems and have seen beloved pets fall sick after presumed exposures to toxicants associated with gas drilling. The levels of proof in each case vary, but the common threads are the types of symptoms and when they occur. These are all people who value living in a small town or country environment, with peacefulness and clean air and water. They have all seen their quiet lives changed drastically. Their passionate, and sometimes eloquent, responses to their troubles inspire us to work harder to understand what has happened to them and to so many like them.

TWO

SARAH AND JOSIE
Violated Families

Do you know what my little girl said? She dreamed that the
guards were gone, the gate, the ropes, and the bright lights
and the noise—all gone, and the hill back to normal, just
being a hill. She just wants this all back to what it was before.
We just want our lives back, the way they were before.
—Sarah Valdes, February 2011

In the rolling hills south of Pittsburgh, the quiet, rural landscape has
undergone a remarkable transformation. Home to many new drilling
sites in recent years, the area has seen truck traffic increase dramatically.
Processing plants, compressor stations, condensate tanks, wastewater
impoundments, drilling-muds pits, and drilling rigs now adorn fields
that were once primarily agricultural land. The change has brought
prosperity for a few landowners and for proprietors of fast-food estab-
lishments, but has been less than beneficial to the many who were unwittingly made victims. This is illustrated dramatically by the plight of
two neighbors, Sarah and Josie, their families, and their animals.

I first received both Sarah Valdes's and Josie Bidermann's names,
along with others, from a former employee of a gas company. After I was
given Sarah's contact information, I was asked not to call her until after
the holidays were over. She was having a tough time with sick animals
and a child who was severely ill, and because of that, the holiday season
would be especially difficult for her.

I was working on another case when my contact called and asked me
to drop everything and phone Josie. It was late, and as I listened to the

prerecorded message after dialing her number and prepared to leave a message, she picked up. She was expecting my call and wanted to tell me everything about her experiences with the gas drilling company, her water problems, and, most importantly, what happened to her dogs and horses.

Josie and her daughter, Lindsay, compete in rodeo and barrel-racing events, keeping their horses in a stable on their farm. Along with Josie's husband, Jeff, they raise dogs—purebred boxers and bulldogs, some of the best in Pennsylvania. These are not city folks playing at being plantation owners, but salt-of-the-earth farmers with a real connection to the land. Jeff has lived in this neighborhood all of his life and was raised by grandparents in their home, a 200-year-old farmhouse on land where beef cattle and pigs were kept and fruit was produced. Josie has lived here only thirty-three years and considers herself an outsider because many of their neighbors, like Jeff, have families that have lived here for generations. To Josie and Jeff, the politics of Harrisburg and Washington, DC, could be happening on another planet. Yet deals were being made with multinational corporations, and their beloved Pennsylvania landscape was being sold to the highest bidder with little or no accountability. On Josie's farm, these deals meant nothing. Protecting the health and welfare of her family and animals was most important.

In the last couple of years, the drilling company had cleared several acres of farmland on the property of her neighbor, Mr. Leverkuhn. Seemingly overnight, this bucolic landscape was transformed into an industrial zone with the arrival of a shale gas well pad situated on higher ground and within a half mile of both Josie's and Sarah's homes. This was soon followed by three wells. Along with the gas wells came a drilling-muds pit that held the drill cuttings, muds, and fluids; an impoundment nearly five acres in size to hold wastewater; and condensate tanks to store semiliquid hydrocarbons that are often produced along with the gas.

As with most landowners, Mr. Leverkuhn was probably unaware of the massive changes that would take place on his land. The landsmen charged with signing up farmers for leases apparently have a rather casual relationship with the truth: rarely is the process of fracking and its potential impacts explained to the landowner—the enticement is monetary, information is secondary. Since even landowners are kept in the dark before signing a lease, neighbors who will have their lives turned upside down are typically unaware of the changes to come. I wonder now, in retrospect, if Mr. Leverkuhn was aware of the dozen or so springs on his property before he leased his land. I wonder if he was aware that the site chosen for development was a recharge area, where surface waters move downward to refill the springs and groundwater that are used by him and his neighbors, including Josie and Sarah, as their sole source of water. And, I wonder, if he knew what he knows now, a few years after drilling began, would he lease again?

While on a tour of her neighborhood, Josie confirmed what I had suspected after having spoken with her by phone for over a year and a half: she worked from her home, her life and business revolved around her animals, and to put it mildly, she was devoted to them. Although she was the type of person who kept to herself and didn't know the neighbors as well as her husband did, Josie admitted, "If it's horse people or dog people, you can ask me [about them] and I'll know them." Josie was also exceptional in that she had a record of every event, every phone call, every meeting that had anything to do with the invaders who had taken over her neighborhood. She was probably the only person I spoke with who knew the distances from her water well to the well pad and wastewater impoundment, from her spring to the well pad and wastewater impoundment, from the well pad to her property line. She had dates corresponding to when the wells were drilled and completed, and when the wastewater impoundment was completed. This last date—the spring of 2010, approximately a year before I first spoke to her—was seared into her brain, because soon after the completion of the impoundment, she lost her well water completely and her spring water dropped to a trickle.

Amazed by Josie's organization, I wondered, if I were to take her place, would I be this organized? Would I be able to cope with bad water, sick and dying animals, and my water service being cut off? (Just before I first spoke with her, the drilling company informed Josie that her water service would be stopped.) Amazingly, Josie and her family soldiered on. When the water well first dried up, Jeff diverted the spring to run into the house. This helped until the spring all but stopped a few months after the wastewater impoundment was completed, at which time Jeff and Josie started hauling water from a nearby creek—325 gallons at a time. It was hard work, but Josie assured me they had to do it. They needed water to wash clothes, wash dishes, take showers, flush the toilets—all things we take for granted. And their horses needed water too. They bought bottled water for themselves and their dogs but couldn't afford it for their horses.

In September 2010, after Josie complained to the drilling company that her spring had been running low since June, the company supplied her family with water temporarily and paid for a new water well to be drilled. While there was no admission that its drilling activities on Mr. Leverkuhn's property caused Josie's water problems, the drilling company did determine that the construction of the impoundment may have inadvertently affected the drainage of Josie's spring water. But her horses were still drinking what little water could be obtained from the spring and whatever the family could haul from the creek. I heard deep guilt in Josie's voice when she talked about her horses. She was speaking with a veterinarian, and she was feeling bad about shortchanging the horses, these animals she loved, these animals that, along with the dogs, were always taken care of first.

Of course I understood, but I had to ask a question, a question she knew was coming: "So your family and your dogs are doing better off the water, but how are your horses doing?"

There was a long pause.

"One has diarrhea. It's not good, but it would be worse if we weren't cutting what's left of the spring water with what we're hauling. I have a barn full of horses—we could never afford to give them bottled water, and we can't physically haul all the water they need." We both agreed she was doing the best she could, better than most people, given the situation, and that it could be much worse. We moved on.

Although she could not afford a full analysis of what was killing her animals, she did have some basic diagnostic tests done. I was interested in the results of these tests in order to understand what happened. The first animal to die after drilling began was Mr. Higgins, Josie's young boxer that served as a stud for her breeding business. By the time I began researching this case, the veterinarian had decided that he was not going to speak to anyone concerning the death of Mr. Higgins. The fact that Josie had given me written permission to obtain all records from him made no difference; he was not talking, and that meant I was cut off from speaking with the first veterinarian who saw Mr. Higgins on emergency.

But after examining Mr. Higgins's medical records, which were graciously supplied by Josie, I could tell that this vet had conducted a complete exam and given Mr. Higgins a presumptive diagnosis of kidney failure with an increased level of calcium. As one of Mr. Higgins's lymph nodes was also mildly enlarged, I agreed that a needle biopsy of this lymph node was a good idea to rule out the possibility of lymphoma, something that wasn't uncommon in this breed. I also knew that because of the progression of the signs and the history, poisoning was a very real possibility.

After reading all of this in the record, why was I being so persistent in wanting to talk to this veterinarian? Simply because I wasn't there to examine Mr. Higgins—I didn't have a chance to see the color of his gums, to pinch his skin to see just how dehydrated he was, to palpate his abdomen and lymph nodes, to listen to his heart and lungs. In short, I didn't see him. Her veterinarian did. He became my eyes, ears, and hands. I needed to talk to him.

Unfortunately, the needle biopsy was never done. Josie grew impatient and brought Mr. Higgins to a specialty clinic where he was given a poor prognosis based mostly on his breed. Josie declined further diagnostics and opted for euthanasia as Mr. Higgins had deteriorated so rapidly, was weak, and could not rise. She couldn't bear to watch him suffer any longer.

What happened here? A young dog, less than two years old, progressed from healthy to incapacitated in a few days, with lab work indicating the possibility of cancer, but also liver and kidney toxicity. Poisoning was suspected. Two days before Mr. Higgins became ill, Josie recalled that a truck had spread wastewater on her road, and Mr. Higgins had lapped up a puddle at the end of the driveway, splashing and playing before she could call him back. What was he exposed to? Josie will never know for sure, but very likely Mr. Higgins drank a cocktail of heavy metals and radioactive and organic compounds that tasted salty and made him want to consume more.

That night, after hearing Josie's story, I thought about my dog, Frankie, also two years old, also euthanized because I couldn't bear to watch him suffer any longer. I thought about how hard that was, but it was a clear-cut decision compared to what Josie had to do. Frankie had uncontrolled idiopathic epilepsy, with increasingly frequent periods of status epilepticus (a prolonged seizure). It was the hardest thing I ever had to do, cut a young dog down like that, yet it was nothing compared to what Josie had endured.

And that should be the end of the story—Josie should not have had to deal with anything else, particularly with the prospect of losing more animals suddenly and without a definitive diagnosis.

During a recent conversation at her home, Josie showed me a trophy case honoring her favorite barrel racer, trained and ridden by Lindsay. "This is Amy. She was pretty special. She gave her heart to Lindsay." Up to now, I had been impressed by how calm Josie had been while describing some of her family's health problems—headaches, nosebleeds, rashes, gastrointestinal upset, severe fatigue, difficulty breathing and concentrating—and even those of her dogs since drilling operations began at Mr. Leverkuhn's site. But while standing in front of this trophy case, she broke down. "It's true, when you have a [horse with a] heart that gives heart, there's not enough money in the world that could ever replace that horse. We turned down sixty thousand dollars for her the year before she died. All we wanted was a baby out of her. And this is Lindsay." She pointed to a picture of a young woman, hair flowing, atop a quarter horse cutting sharply around a barrel, girl and horse moving as one. There were many trophies—several dozen. Josie was weeping quietly. "Year after year, grand champions with everything. When we bought Amy, she was a six-month-old baby. I traded a sixty-five-hundred-dollar horse and two thousand in cash for a six-month-old baby that I never . . . I just said, 'I'm crazy. I would never spend this for a six-month-old baby.' And my daughter said, 'Mom, I see things in her. I want her.'" Josie paused and turned to look at me. "She was right. She knew. And that horse, when she broke her leg, they weren't sure that she'd ever come back to racing. We kept her in a cast. We kept her in a hoist. Lindsay went down there umpteen times a day: before school, after school, before going to bed. We swam her three days a week for almost three months—that's how Lindsay exercised her. And see what she came back and she did?" Josie asked. "So you tell me, that horse didn't have heart?"

Less than three months after Mr. Higgins's death, Amy had a veterinary examination and was pronounced healthy. A few weeks later, however, she stopped eating and began to lose weight, appearing off-balance and uncoordinated. The veterinarian thought that Amy might have an infection, and treated her with steroids, antibiotics, and antihistamines. Two days later, Amy was still not eating, and her balance problem was worse. Not certain what to do at this point, the veterinarian treated Amy for a neurological disease called equine protozoal myeloencephalitis. This disease is difficult to diagnose, but seemed to be a reasonable guess at the time. Three days later, Amy was no better. Alarmed, Josie called the veterinarian again. This time, when he came out, he treated Amy again and took blood for testing. Two days later, Amy's back legs became so weak that it was difficult for her to stand. Unable to rise, she sunk down in her stall and began convulsing. Two weeks after she stopped eating, Amy was euthanized. Blood results received after Amy was euthanized indicated liver failure due to toxicity. Josie's veterinarian suspected poisoning, possibly from heavy metals, but the illness remained undiagnosed because neither a necropsy nor further tests were done. Again Josie was forced to choose euthanasia so as not to watch a beloved pet suffer. And again, not knowing why.

Was the drilling company watching? According to Josie, representatives of the company appeared on the scene soon after Amy was euthanized and offered to do the neighborly thing—haul Amy away to be incinerated. In a more perfect world, Josie would have been able to afford having Amy necropsied and tested for toxins in her body, in particular her liver, to see what actually killed her. This is also true for Mr. Higgins. But those sorts of tests are quite expensive, and Josie was not in a position to have them done.

This behavior on the part of a drilling company was apparently not uncommon, as I had heard the same scenario from other animal owners living in intensively drilled areas. It left me with more questions than answers. For example, why isn't the drilling company keeping its workers busy with drilling-related work rather than PR work? Certainly it takes time and energy to be aware of which animals are dying where and under what circumstances. More importantly, if the drilling company really wanted to be a good neighbor, as it liked to portray itself in the media, why didn't it offer to pay for Amy's necropsy and further testing to determine a cause of death, which could easily have cost more than $2,000? Coming on the scene at just the right moment and offering to haul potential evidence away might be perceived by some people as an admission of guilt. If unconventional gas drilling is perfectly safe and there is absolutely no reason to believe that it could possibly be associated with the death of an animal, why wouldn't the drilling company offer to help an animal owner who not only lost her water, but was also losing her animals, her own health, and the health of her family? After all, what could it possibly have to lose?

Not long after speaking to Josie, I called her neighbor, Sarah Valdes, the single mom who was a nurse, the woman with the sick child who I had been warned not to call during the holidays. Two women in the same neighborhood, dealing with the same general trauma, but each was coping completely differently. Where Josie funneled her energies into recording and keeping exact information, Sarah poured her heart into endless patience and maintaining calm for the sake of her children— Patty, who was ten, and David, who was thirteen.

Sarah lived in a farmhouse she estimated as being well over one hundred years old and owned by her extended family for most of that time. She bought it in 1999, just before Patty was born, and lived there for over thirteen years, remodeling the house from top to bottom, with plans to replace the barn. "It was a beautiful place to be, to raise my kids," Sarah said. "We had such a good life there. They had everything they could ever want. It was the perfect location. But it's gone. That's what I tell the kids. It was just a house."

Now face-to-face, I asked the questions I usually held until the end, that I had been waiting to ask since our first conversation more than eighteen months ago, and now, after hearing how good life was before drilling started, needed to ask even more: Why did you sign a lease with the drilling company? And why did you convince Josie and another neighbor to sign with you?

Her answers surprised me, caught me completely off guard, and again made me realize that each person's situation was unique.

"I was afraid of losing my water because we've always had to haul our own water." She pointed across the street from where we sat in the rental house, to her parents' home—where there was no water well and, until very recently, no municipal water—where she'd helped to haul water ever since she could remember. "That farmhouse was the first place I ever lived in that had water. We had an abundant supply of water. We could wash dishes, take showers, wash our vehicles, do laundry, and never had to worry about running out of water." The water was so good and so plentiful, Sarah said, that she shared it with her parents and her church.

Ironically, Sarah, Josie, and another neighbor had all heard about water contamination associated with unconventional gas drilling before signing no-drill leases (no surface drilling or drill sites permitted on the leased premises) in 2007. But they decided to lease as a group and protect themselves with an added clause guaranteeing that if there were any problems with their water supply, the gas drilling company would supply them with water.

"And thank God we added that clause because people around us that didn't do that, they've had a really hard time [obtaining water]. But it didn't help us with the air. We had no idea about that part."

During a tour of her neighborhood in August 2012, Sarah described her road before it was paved: "It was a dirt road, and I took a picture of a tanker truck going down the road. There was a car between me and the truck, and you couldn't even see it [the car] because the dust was so bad." This was back in the beginning, when Sarah and her family were trying to live in their house situated just off the road, trying to adapt to the dust, the dirt, and the noise caused by the constant drilling traffic.

The deteriorating road and the dust took a toll on her car, too, as she has had numerous flat tires, a cracked rim, and a broken air conditioner.

I'd heard a lot about this house, this road, this neighborhood, and I was in the middle of asking more questions, when Sarah told me to slow my car down and stop. A large pad appeared just off the road—approximately five miles from her previous house. We were a few hundred feet away, but with a clear view of the entire pad, the first one I've seen from the road where there were no obstructions. To the left, there were seven wellheads, each appearing as a blue cross connected by a yellow shroud. On the right side of the pad, there were many green tanks—some shaped like long torpedoes, others like giant soup cans—and several silver cylinders connected to what appeared to be smokestacks. These wells are in production, Sarah explained, with pipelines running over the hill behind the pad and to a nearby compressor station.

As we drove away, Sarah spoke about the house again—how difficult it is to keep up with both rental and mortgage payments. We passed many well pads on the way to her previous home, but because most are at the end of no-trespass access roads, there wasn't much to see. Along a beautiful ridge, on a narrow paved and curvy road, Sarah's house huddled off the side at the end of a steep, short driveway. I noticed the barn first, behind and to the left of the house. I envisioned all the animals Patty and David had cared for and raised here—the pigs, rabbits, goats, chickens, cats, dogs, horses and a donkey. I spied what looked like a hutch, but Sarah told me that it was the chicken coop, and that the rabbit pens were just beyond.

"My friend wanted to build a chicken coop," Sarah said, "and I said, 'Come and get it!' My barn was falling down—it had stalls in there. That's where we kept the goats and pigs, and behind it was a lean-to, for the horses. I was planning on building a barn." But after what happened, she's glad she never put the money into that.

Sarah led the way to the house along a stone walkway surrounded by an overgrown lawn. She was embarrassed that the grass hadn't been mowed, but it's difficult to maintain the lawn when just being here makes her ill. Before climbing the steps to the porch, I turned to take in the view—it was gorgeous—across the valley to the next ridge, and because the neighbors are spread out along this road, the house gave the feeling of privacy and seclusion. The porch was big and had once been filled with furniture, now donated to a friend. A trumpet vine was growing wild, but Sarah used to weave it in and out of the railings every spring and summer. From the outside, this two-story home appeared to be in good shape, especially for one not currently lived in. In addition to the unkempt yard, the only indication that something had gone terribly wrong here was the presence of the water buffalo in the back, provided by the drilling company nearly two years ago.

Sarah unlocked the door, and the odor hit us before we could even step in. "What is that smell?" I asked. Sarah said she didn't know. It wasn't an old or closed-in house smell—I couldn't put my finger on it, but I was hoping that I could figure this out before we left. I knew Sarah lost her sense of smell at one point, and now I asked her if it had returned. "Yes," she said. "It's back. There, for a while, I couldn't smell. We would be here, and we wouldn't be able to smell it. The week before we left, my girlfriend was here trying to help me move, and she could smell a horrible odor, and none of us could smell it. After being away, I can smell it."

We walked through a spacious kitchen and peered into the family room. Toys, boxes, pillows, and assorted household items were strewn everywhere, left behind in the rush to move out. "Part of me wants to come and sort through things," Sarah said, "and part of me doesn't even want to be bothered." We climbed a narrow staircase to the second floor, where David's room was the first to greet us. I stepped in, looking out the window from his room, the bedroom closest to Mr. Leverkuhn's wastewater impoundment. I imagined being a child in this room, with the window open, the breeze coming off the impoundment. Sarah said that she didn't know if that had made it worse for her son.

She asked if I'd seen the pictures of the impoundment from Google Earth. Yes, I had, and I had also seen the aerators in the impoundment. From the aerial photos, the aerators look like fountains spread on a large rectangular lagoon, misting whatever was in the wastewater into the air. Then with a mother's guilt, Sarah admitted, "We didn't even know it [the impoundment] was up there until after we figured out what was going on. We just thought it was a well pad."

While still upstairs, Sarah mentioned that her great-grandfather lived in this house many years ago while her father was growing up and that when she first moved in, she planned to finish the trim in the house when the children were older. Now, it's another thing that will never happen. I sensed sadness in her voice, for she had meant to be loyal to this house, to her father and great-grandfather.

Less than ten minutes inside her house, Sarah developed a metal taste in her mouth, which forced us to leave sooner than I'd have liked. "I knew I had a [metal] taste in my mouth," she said, "but I didn't realize how bad it was until we went to New York City for five days. It went away completely." The irony of leaving her home in the countryside and feeling better after staying in a big city for a few days was not lost on Sarah. When she returned home, the taste in her mouth returned too. "If I stay here, it will come back," she said. "We were here for a short while a few weeks ago, and I had it the rest of the day and into the next day."

On the way out, we passed through the kitchen again, which Sarah had remodeled eight years ago. It's large and open, windows facing out to the back with a wood stove with inlaid cherry behind and above the stove. It means a lot to her, this woodwork, made by her father from a cherry tree cut down on her grandfather's farm years ago. But to remove it would be difficult as the cherry was literally set in stone. Just past the woodstove, there was a cupboard, partly open and full of canned and bagged goods. When I noticed the wine, Sarah said it was homemade and that she knew she should take it. "I canned, and we always had our own meat, our own chickens, our own eggs. I come over here to work, and I can't stay for more than half hour to forty-five minutes. I start getting sick—I get a headache."

She described how the air here used to be much worse. "The air is not as heavy now. There were times when I would come over in the morning—the air would feel dewy. You could just feel the chemicals on you. I would just try to get from the car into the house. It was so thick. It's almost like a bug that is caught in a fogger. Now I know what a bug must feel like. I felt like I couldn't breathe—I would get so short of breath."

Air tests were done on Sarah's and Josie's properties in October 2011 through a nonprofit organization that provides testing to low-

income families that have been affected by industrial drilling operations. The results confirmed the miasmic atmosphere that once surrounded the two women's homes, the list of detected chemicals reading
like an environmentalist's worst nightmare: BTEX (benzene, toluene,
ethylbenzene, m-xylene, p-xylene, and o-xylene); carbon tetrachloride;
chloromethane; methylene chloride; tetrachloroethylene; trichlorofluoromethane; 1,1,2-trichloro-1,2,2-trifluoroethane; and 1,2,4-trimeth-
ylbenzene.

As we pulled out of the driveway and back on to this precariously
narrow road, I stopped to look across the valley one last time. "If the
leaves were off," Sarah said, "you'd have a direct view of [Mr.
Leverkuhn's] impoundment."

On Mr. Leverkuhn's property, the first unconventional gas well was
drilled in September 2009, and a few months later, the process of horizontal high-volume hydraulic fracturing on this well was completed.
Within several years, three gas wells would occupy Mr. Leverkuhn's
land. The chemicals pumped down to hydraulically fracture the first
well fell under five broad categories: friction reducer, bactericide, gell-
ing agent, oxygen scavenger, and scale inhibitor. As I paged through the
material safety data sheets for these chemicals, I noticed that several
were proprietary mixes, meaning that only some of the chemicals making up these blends were listed. Exactly what percentage was listed varied with the mix. For example, FRW-200,[1] the friction reducer, was
made up of 17.6 to 26 percent petroleum distillates, the remaining 74 to
82.4 percent of the ingredients were anyone's guess. Could some of
these chemicals escape the cement casing and make their way into Mr.
Leverkuhn's and his neighbors' groundwater? According to a recent
survey of leaking Marcellus Shale gas wells in Pennsylvania from 2010
to 2012,[2] approximately 6 to 7 percent were reported to have cement
casings with compromised structural integrity during the first year,
which is consistent with data from the US Mineral Management Service
showing similar failure rates for cement jobs leading to "sustained casing pressure" for wells drilled in the Gulf of Mexico, cited earlier.[3]

Unfortunately, numerous spills and leaks occurred on Mr. Leverkuhn's property in 2010 and 2011, risking contamination of his and his

neighbors' water sources; in most cases, neither Josie nor Sarah were aware of these events until much later. Some of these occurrences involved the transfer of drilling fluids and wastewater between Mr. Leverkuhn's site and other nearby sites via tanker trucks. In one case, drilling muds leaked and were spilled during transfer from tanks to trucks, and several other times, spills of wastewater occurred including discharge outside the impoundment during offloading. In another incident, diesel fuel and wastewater spilled during a transfer between trucks, and on a separate occasion, several hundred gallons of wastewater splashed from tanks onto the ground because debris blocked the outflow. Several incidents stand out in Josie and Sarah's memory—the time wastewater spilled when a tanker truck overturned on Mr. Leverkuhn's snow-covered access road, and another time, when a driver left a valve open and wastewater spilled from the truck, running down the access road and onto the public road before entering Mr. Leverkuhn's cow pasture.

In addition to transferring fluids using tanker trucks, the drilling company operating on Mr. Leverkuhn's land also moved fluids using temporary plastic pipelines that may course for miles on the ground. During transfers, pipes can crack and leak due to freezing and thawing or when fluids are run through the pipes at pressures higher than the pipes are rated to handle. During 2010 and 2011, several leaks associated with Mr. Leverkuhn's site occurred during pipeline transfers of fracturing fluid and wastewater. In December 2010, a leak occurred directly on the Leverkuhn well site in a line carrying fracturing fluid. A few weeks before this leak was observed, lines were discovered leaking fracturing fluid and wastewater in three separate places between Mr. Leverkuhn's well pad and another pad located approximately a mile away. Soon after these discoveries, several more leaks occurred when air-release valves and drain valves malfunctioned in lines transferring wastewater between Mr. Leverkuhn's pad and another pad located over a mile away. At the end of January 2011, yet another wastewater leak in a transfer line occurred between these same two well sites.

On the Leverkuhn site, both the wastewater impoundment and the drilling-muds pit were open to the air above them, but below, two liners were supposed to separate the ground from the chemical-fluid mix that would eventually fill both depressions. The problem with liners is that they can rip and tear anytime, even during installation; this happened at Mr. Leverkuhn's impoundment on several occasions. Wildlife, caught off guard while encountering pits and impoundments on well pad sites, often become entrapped and have to be removed,[4] even after fencing has been placed. Two deer were found in Mr. Leverkuhn's impoundment in May 2010, along with tears in the liner, presumably from their attempts to escape, and at the drilling-muds pit, a fox was discovered clawing and biting the pit liner after becoming trapped in early November 2010. Just three weeks later, after repairs had been made to the pit liner, another fox created more holes while attempting to escape.

The first sign of a problem with the drilling-muds pit liner wasn't revealed until an inspection in March 2010, where a leak that smelled of sewage water was reported seeping from the slope of the pad and within three hundred feet of one of Mr. Leverkuhn's springs. Soon after, the contents of the pit were analyzed and found to contain drilling-related substituents, several of which were later detected in both Josie's and Sarah's water. From then on, the drilling-muds pit lived a troubled life. It would be rebuilt and relined in May 2010. It would be used to hold the drill cuttings, muds, and fluids from two more wells drilled on Mr. Leverkuhn's property in January 2011. In May 2011, after water results indicated significant changes in both Mr. Leverkuhn's upper spring (used for potable water) and his lower spring (used for livestock) since drilling operations began, the drilling company graciously provided a water buffalo to his family. But a suspicious eye was cast upon the drilling-muds pit. Over the coming months, the Leverkuhn pit liner would be removed and the pit would be purged of seven hundred tons of drill cuttings and fourteen hundred tons of contaminated soil and flushed with thirty thousand gallons of water before chloride levels returned to background (what they were before drilling began) and sodium levels dropped dramatically but still remained approximately twice that of background levels. The final death knell for the pit occurred in April 2012, when the company submitted plans for permanent closure, which eventually occurred in the fall of 2012.

Like the pit, the Leverkuhn impoundment did not live a carefree life. In fact, one could say that it started its life on the wrong foot. Leak detection systems on centralized impoundments using two-liner systems such as Mr. Leverkuhn's must be placed *between* the two liners, according to Pennsylvania law.[5] In theory, this would allow leaks to be detected before reaching any surface or ground water. By placing the leak detection system *underneath* both liners, any leakage of the contents within the impoundment was more likely to cause contamination of water sources before detection, which is apparently what happened at the Leverkuhn impoundment. Comparison of water analyses on the fluids in the impoundment and the leak detection system demonstrated that the impoundment was leaking from November 2010 to May 2012 and possibly months before. As of May 2013, the fate of the impoundment had not yet been determined, but it is under investigation to determine the extent of any contamination and any remediation that may follow.

In July 2010, soon after the wastewater impoundment was completed, both Josie and Sarah noticed a rotten-egg or raw-sewage odor in the air around their properties. Suspecting that this odor might be hydrogen sulfide and related to the activities at Mr. Leverkuhn's site, they promptly complained to the drilling company and the PADEP. Hydrogen sulfide is a poisonous, colorless gas that often accompanies methane gas as it returns to the surface, and could also be produced by bacteria in wastewater impoundments;[6] it has a tendency to cause health problems in people living near gas drilling operations, specifically causing signs of respiratory distress and neurological effects such as incoordination, headaches, impaired memory, and loss of the sense of smell.[7] Over the next few months, in an effort to reduce the odors, the drilling company treated the wastewater impoundment on Mr. Leverkuhn's land with two biocides, acrolein and MC B-8642 (a mix that is 30 to 60 percent glutaraldehyde).[8] Both chemicals may cause severe irritation to the eyes, skin, and respiratory tract.[9]

Large impoundments such as Mr. Leverkuhn's often have aerators to decrease odors as well as to increase evaporation by misting the fluid into the air. The bacteria that produce the chemical compounds that give off the sulfur smell are anaerobic—that is, they live under conditions of low or no oxygen. One of the reasons that the aerators are installed is to inhibit the growth of these bacteria. During the time the impoundment was treated with acrolein and glutaraldehyde, additional aerators were installed, increasing the likelihood that toxic chemicals would be dispersed into the air. And because the chemicals are often heavier than air, these actions increased the chances that neighbors such as Josie and Sarah and their animals, living nearby and at lower elevations, would be inhaling the toxins coming off Mr. Leverkuhn's impoundment.

Soon after drilling began on the first unconventional gas well on Mr. Leverkuhn's property in September 2009, Sarah's son David became ill with nondescript stomach pain, backache, and sore throat. Although the whole family would experience unusual illness over the coming months in the form of headaches, nosebleeds, rashes, fatigue, and gastrointestinal upset, it was David who was hit the hardest and seemed the least able to fight off whatever it was that was making the whole family sick.

When I spoke to Sarah for the first time, in February 2011, I didn't learn how devastating her son's illness was. Sarah wanted me to first understand what had happened to the animals—hers and Josie's—and she wanted answers on how and why these animals died. She was very patient with my questions but very persistent, even though she was exhausted; the only time we could talk was after Patty and David were fed and in bed, and all the animal chores were done. Again, as with Josie, I asked myself, how does this woman cope? Two sick children, water gone bad, and facing it all as a single working mom—this situation seemed even more overwhelming than Josie's because Sarah was going it alone.

I asked Sarah if her water level had dropped like Josie's had. No, she said, but she wished it had—then they would have stopped drinking it. Sarah's family initially continued to drink the water because the changes, such as a faint odor, were so subtle at first. But when the smell worsened and the sediment became obvious, they stopped drinking the water altogether but continued to use it for bathing, dishes, and laundry. Later, Sarah felt as guilty about giving her children the well water to drink and use as Josie felt about giving her horses the spring water.

Sarah mentioned Mr. Higgins and asked whether Josie had told me about David's dog, Quinn. It was very likely that both dogs were poisoned by wastewater—Mr. Higgins after drinking from a puddle at the end of Josie's driveway, and Quinn after running around Mr. Leverkuhn's well pad and being exposed to the runoff from the well site and directly from the impoundment, which at that time was not fenced off. Surely enough animals had died, but Sarah still wasn't telling me what happened to David. Was there more?

As I would soon learn, Josie, as a part of her dog-breeding business, was caring for pregnant animals at this time. Her boxer bitch, Bessie, experienced dystocia[10] and lost two puppies at term. One was born with a cleft palate and died the same day, and another was stillborn. Josie was unprepared for this because Bessie was in good health up to and during the pregnancy, and she had whelped three healthy litters before this. It would take a fifth litter and the loss of fifteen pups (seven stillborn and eight dead within a day, all the pups afflicted with congenital hypotrichosis, that is, they were born with the complete or partial absence of normal hair) before Josie moved her dogs to the homes of friends and family who lived in parts of Pennsylvania that still had clean air and water.

By November 2010, Josie and Sarah had lost animals, had lost their water, and were beginning to suspect that they were losing their air. Maybe it took the loss of this many beloved pets, dying mysteriously, for Sarah to make the vital connection between what was happening to them and what was happening to her son.

Then she told her doctor about it.

By then, David had been in and out of the hospital and had missed approximately a year of school, innumerable hours in after-school clubs and sports, and time with his friends. He'd missed more than he could ever think about. He was fourteen and a half, nearly fifteen, and he was more familiar with his mom's nurse friends than he was with his own friends. Essentially he was missing being a teenager. And all because his doctor couldn't figure out what was wrong with him. The tests that were run—the complete blood count, the strep throat screen, the Epstein Barr virus AB panel—gave no answers. On hearing what had been happening to the animals in Sarah's neighborhood, David's doctor snapped into action, ordering many basic tests (again) but also a screen to look for heavy metals—including thallium, cobalt, mercury, cadmium, lead, and arsenic—in David's urine.

On David's medical report, arsenic was the last metal listed, but it was in boldface. Across from this entry, a few inches over and also in boldface, were the words "85 micrograms/gram" next to an *H*, also in bold, for "high." The report also included a biological exposure index, a reference value that is used by engineers, industrial hygienists, nurses, and physicians to help assess and prevent injury of industrial workers exposed to chemicals.[11]

But David wasn't an industrial worker.

If he worked in the metal smelting, glass manufacturing, microelectronics, or semiconductor industry, then his high level of arsenic would be understandable. But he was just a teenager who happened to live next to an industrial gas drilling operation. He was being poisoned. And Sarah could not do anything about it. She hired a hydrogeologist and a toxicologist. Over the next months, she would spend thousands of dollars on water tests and consultations. She would spend countless hours in the hospital with Patty and David while the whole family was tested. They would lug around jugs for twenty-four-hour urine samples. They were living a nightmare. These were the things they had to do—were expected to do—if there was any hope of escape.

In early November 2010, Josie and Sarah filed complaints of poor water quality with the drilling company and the PADEP. This was not the first time the women had taken this course of action, but now the message was stronger because both families were suffering from many of the same symptoms observed in people living near gas drilling operations around the country: headaches; nosebleeds; burning of the eyes, nose, and throat; rashes; severe and debilitating fatigue; and gastrointestinal symptoms, including nausea, vomiting, and diarrhea. And their complaints held a special urgency because in both cases, otherwise healthy animals had been lost coincidentally and suddenly, since the onset of drilling operations.

This time, their requests were taken seriously and the drilling company arranged for testing of their water sources. Ideally, their water should have been tested *before* gas drilling operations ever began on Mr. Leverkuhn's land; without predrill testing, it is difficult to know if contaminants detected later were present initially. But Pennsylvania Act 13,[12] which would require drilling companies to offer predrill water

testing to all Pennsylvania residents within twenty-five hundred feet of
a proposed wellhead, hadn't yet been passed; in 2009, when operations
were ramping up on Mr. Leverkuhn's land, the law only required testing
to be offered to those residents within a thousand feet of a proposed gas
well. As Josie lived just beyond one thousand feet, and Sarah even further, their water had never been tested.

As would later be determined by a consulting hydrogeologist, both
Josie and Sarah shared the same water table as Mr. Leverkuhn's pad site,
as well as a neighbor who lived, like them, downgradient from the site
(that is, the groundwater flows down from the pad site to the homes),
and Mr. Leverkuhn, who lived upgradient from the well pad named after him (that is, the groundwater flows from his home to the well pad).
In light of the leaking that occurred from Mr. Leverkuhn's impoundment into the groundwater they all depended on, the shared aquifer was
certainly not good news for anyone's drinking water. However, because
predrill testing was done on these neighbors' water sources, their samples could serve as a baseline for both Josie and Sarah. It came as no
surprise to either woman that these predrill water tests indicated no
significant contamination.

Because the drilling company had recently drilled a replacement
water well for Josie's family in October 2010, this well was tested along
with her spring water in November 2010. Sarah's spring and well water
were also tested in November 2010, and pending results of the water
tests, the drilling company provided Sarah's family with a water buffalo
at this time. While a long list of unsavory chemicals was detected in the
water sources of each family, many were the same. These included fracturing fluid additives such as ethylene glycol, propylene glycol, ethanol,
butanol, and propanol.[13] They included the trihalomethanes such as
chloroform, bromodichloromethane, and dibromochloromethane, all
considered carcinogens and all uncommon detects in unchlorinated private water sources such as Josie's and Sarah's.[14]

Mr. Leverkuhn's wastewater impoundment and its leak detection
system, also known as the manhole, were also tested at the same time
that Josie's and Sarah's water sources were tested, in November 2010.
The first set of tests done on the manhole and the wastewater impoundment on November 10 signaled that both sources had similar levels of

minerals and heavy metals such as chloride, barium, iron, manganese, sodium, and strontium as well as fracturing fluid additives, including propylene glycol and surfactants. That both the manhole and the impoundment had similar levels of these chemicals positively indicated that the impoundment was leaking or had been leaking for some time. Repeat testing done on November 19 confirmed not only that the impoundment was leaking, but also that the leak was worsening.

In short, the chemicals detected in both Josie's and Sarah's water sources clearly represented what one would expect from water contaminated by a nearby unconventional gas drilling operation. In particular, several chemicals leaking from Mr. Leverkuhn's wastewater impoundment were also detected in Josie's and Sarah's water sources; these chemicals included propylene glycol, propanol, and ammonia. And as stated above, several chemicals detected in Mr. Leverkuhn's drilling-muds pit following a liner leak were later observed in Josie's and Sarah's water sources and included barium, chromium, 1,3,5-trimethylbenzene, ammonia, oil, and grease.

Nevertheless, after reviewing the water results, the drilling company sent letters to both Josie and Sarah in January 2011, cheerfully pointing to its responsible practices and lack of responsibility for the women's water-quality problems. With concurrence from the PADEP, both families were advised by the drilling company that their water deliveries would soon cease.

David's arsenic level was elevated, but the question on everyone's mind was how it came to be that way. Arsenic levels were negligible in Sarah's water when it was tested, but because no testing was done when David first became ill in the fall of 2009—approximately one year before the water was tested—it is difficult to know exactly what the levels of arsenic may have been in the water just after drilling began.

As a nurse and a mother, Sarah was devastated by not knowing what the long-term health effects of arsenic would be in her children, especially David. She could not run away from this problem, get it fixed, or get it reversed. It meant that her children, because of where she chose to live, might be carrying traces of this poison in their bodies for months. But because children exposed to arsenic may suffer the same health effects as adults—increased risk of bladder, kidney, liver, lung, skin, and prostate cancer[15]—David and Patty might be dealing with its consequences for the rest of their lives.

When Sarah told me this, I thought, haven't these people endured enough?

I was receiving updates from Sarah every month or so, sometimes more often. What happened next, in December 2010, when David's urine was rechecked for heavy metals, was actually good news: David's arsenic level dropped very low and continued to stay below the cutoff—the magic number of fifty micrograms per gram—in the coming months, as did readings on Sarah and Patty. By that time, Sarah had switched to bottled water for drinking and a water buffalo for everything else (washing clothes and dishes, showers, baths, brushing teeth, flushing the toilet) and was providing her animals with drinking water from a water buffalo after the drilling company refused to do so. Things were looking up, and I thought they would just keep heading in that direction. After all, what else could go wrong?

We think of water and air as synonymous with life, yet while we can sometimes change our water supply, we cannot do so with the air we breathe. In some locations, we can switch from well water to city water. In rural areas of Pennsylvania, the only other option besides a well might be a water buffalo. Although inconvenient and expensive, a water buffalo is a choice that can be made for those who can afford it and can temporarily replace a contaminated water supply. But providing a new air supply because the air has become tainted is not practical. Three months after she found out that her son was suffering from arsenic poisoning, Sarah learned that she, Patty, and David tested positive for phenol, which is a metabolite of benzene. David's level was especially worrying, as it was consistent with chronic exposure to benzene at levels of 0.5 to 4.0 parts per million (ppm) in the air. So now it was the air, and another poison. This time, it was benzene, a known carcinogen.

Many volatile organic compounds, including benzene, were escaping Mr. Leverkuhn's wastewater impoundment and entering the air, as would be evidenced by a test done months later. Benzene is everywhere in gas drilling country: drilling companies use it as a component of drill-ing muds and hydraulic fracturing fluid, and it is also found naturally in the layers of shale containing the gas. When the gas comes to the sur-face, benzene comes along with it, eventually being separated from the gas during processing at compressor stations. But it doesn't stop there: benzene is a component of diesel fuel, which is used by compressor sta-tions and the huge trucks that, in drilling country, wallpaper the land-scape and make a simple bicycle ride a life-threatening experience. Nothing can match the thrill of a quiet bike ride periodically inter-rupted by forty-ton trucks speeding by two or three feet from your ear. Worst of all, benzene is extremely volatile—it can escape into the air from any open surface and can vent from leaky condensate tanks. Since it is a component of the wastewater, the sprawling surface area of the impoundment and the action of the aerators pump benzene into the air for miles around. Likewise, benzene that is brought to the surface with drilling fluids, muds, and cuttings and subsequently dumped in pits, also ends up in the air. And benzene is released into the atmosphere when gas wells are flared.

But it didn't end there. David and Patty also had trace levels of hip-puric acid in their urine. When toluene enters the body, it is converted to hippuric acid, so finding hippuric acid in the urine may indicate an exposure to toluene. Now toluene, like benzene, is a volatile organic compound that is a component of diesel and other products used in hydraulic fracturing fluids, and is found in the condensate produced at compressor stations. Also like benzene, it is regulated under the Safe Drinking Water Act (SDWA) and is listed as a hazardous air pollutant under the Clean Air Act.[16] And, like benzene, toluene is a found in the wastewater.

Sarah now wondered how she could continue to live at her home and protect her children and herself. She knew that benzene could cause leukemia and anemia, and that children were particularly susceptible.[17] She also discovered that both benzene and toluene could affect their vi-sion[18] and sense of smell[19] and that toluene could cause loss of hear-ing.[20] But the other symptoms she had read about—the fatigue, sore throat, nosebleeds, nasal and eye irritation, drowsiness, dizziness, nausea, headache, and chemical taste in their mouths—these things they had been dealing with for months. Maybe if she kept the children and the animals inside with the windows closed and play dates scheduled elsewhere? But David and Patty were adolescents, and they desperately missed spending time with their friends in their own rooms, in their own house. Sarah wondered if the drilling company would be a good neighbor and at least pay for air testing.

Sarah sent me a package with photos, medical results, veterinary records, and journal entries, so that I could see what happened when. On the date when she first learned about the phenol in their bodies, she wrote how she and the children had been waiting for these results, and now they know these chemicals are in the air and they are breathing them off the wastewater impoundment. She wrote how upset they are by this news, but concluded the entry with a statement: "Our animals were not tested for these things."

Toxicology testing is very expensive, as stated above, and screening can be tricky because you have to know what you're looking for. Otherwise, it's just an expensive way of searching for a needle in a haystack. None of the animals that died had screens for organic chemicals, and more importantly, the drilling company never provided a full list of what chemicals were used in drilling and fracturing. Nor did it provide a complete analysis of the wastewater.

Two months after initial urine tests showed elevated levels of phenol in David's urine, repeat tests showed dramatic increases in his level as well as that of his mother and sister—all consistent with chronic exposure to benzene at levels of 0.5 to 4.0 ppm in the air. Also, the levels of hippuric acid were dramatically increased for all members of the family.[21]

Sarah thought daily of leaving her home, but she always had the same conclusion: "We can't afford to move, and what about the animals?" What would she do if for some reason they were forced to move? This now seemed her worse nightmare. She tried not to think or talk about it—it was too depressing. It was like being in a bad dream where everything you cherish turns to dust when you touch it. Approximately one and a half years after drilling began, it happened. Her worst nightmare came to life.

There had been a power outage in the neighborhood in May 2011; ironically, it occurred on Mother's Day, and would be something that Sarah would never forget. It lasted only a few hours but caused a cascade of events that would throw Sarah and her children's lives into even more turmoil. Due to the outage, the aerators at the wastewater impoundment stopped working and the impoundment became septic. The odors were much worse than they were a year before, when the impoundment was treated chemically and more aerators were added after Sarah and Josie complained. Now, the odors were similar to walking through the tunnels of a city's sewer, the smell of human feces triggering an irresistible urge to vomit. The weather didn't help, changing from bright and dry to wet and humid, the smell hanging around their neighborhood like a toxic fog.

The physical signs they had been experiencing—headaches, fatigue, nosebleeds, and sore throats—intensified. In Sarah's household, David again suffered the most, sleeping for eighteen hours and having to be dragged from his bed and awakened by Sarah, as if from a drugged sleep. She recalled the health impacts of benzene and toluene: they can affect the nervous system at even low levels, making a person appear drunk and extremely tired. Sarah stayed on, not knowing what else to do. They became nauseated. They lost their sense of smell, but didn't realize it until a friend visited and asked how they could possibly tolerate the stench. Sarah had convinced herself that her family had simply acclimated to the smell, but after her friend visited, she scheduled an appointment with her doctor and learned that she and the children had anosmia—they were losing their sense of smell. Sarah also learned that she was losing her hearing. The doctor advised her and the children to leave their home for at least thirty days—or suffer more severe health consequences.

For Josie, the septic impoundment caused the same problems, but perhaps more intensely because she worked at home and refused to leave her horses. Again she kept careful notes and called the drilling company and the PADEP, reporting that the stench had worsened; it was making her so sick she couldn't function. She made a reasonable request to both the drilling company and the PADEP—to test the air quality. Not only was her request for testing denied by both parties, but the regulatory agency did not cite the drilling company for air pollution. Ignored too many times, Josie decided to force the PADEP to investigate her complaints of water and air pollution in a "complete, scientific and non-arbitrary manner" by seeking a writ of mandamus in June 2011. Such a writ orders a public agency or governmental body to perform an act required by law when it has neglected or refused to do so. Basically, Josie was demanding that the PADEP do its job.

While Josie decided to stay put, Sarah responded by taking her doctor's advice and moved her family out of her home in May 2011. During the time away from their home, Sarah would live out of her car before moving in with a friend and sleeping on a couch. David would stay with a friend from school, and Patty would stay with Sarah's mother. Meanwhile, medical tests would show that phenol and hippuric acid levels in the children were down, and David would continue to have low arsenic levels, but Sarah's phenol levels would remain elevated: her daily trips home to take care of the animals she was forced to leave behind exposed her to the air for one or two hours every day. During this time, the children would beg to go back to the house and visit the animals. Sarah would relent, and after a few visits, David would become so sick that he would have to return to the hospital, with abdominal pain, swollen lymph nodes, and headaches.

But ultimately, for Sarah's family, there was no good solution, no good choice. They were wearing out their welcome staying elsewhere, they missed their friends and their farm, and no place except their own house was big enough to keep the family and all their farm animals and pets together. With the end of the summer of 2011, the approach of the county fair, and the start of school, they moved back. With the family back home less than a week, the symptoms that had disappeared after they left the farm would now return with a vengeance: sore throats, swollen lymph nodes, headaches, nosebleeds, fatigue, the metallic taste in their mouths. And with two compressor stations up and running within one mile from their home, a sickeningly sweet chemical smell permeated the air and exacerbated their symptoms, making them want to vomit. Initially forced to leave because of health issues and forced to return because of economics, they were forced to leave again because of health issues, but this time it would be for good.

.   .   .

The former gas company employee who had originally asked me to contact Sarah and Josie sent me a video of a community meeting in an area that was being intensively drilled.[22] He wanted me to see and hear that Sarah and Josie were not alone in their opinions of the impacts that unconventional gas drilling had on their neighborhood. When I first viewed this video, I assumed it was recorded in their neighborhood because the course of events and the citizens' comments were the same as what I was hearing from Sarah and Josie. It wasn't until I went back to watch the video a second time and transcribe what was said that I noticed that this meeting was recorded in a nearby community, more than a year before the impoundment in Sarah and Josie's neighborhood went septic.

In the video, the meeting is held in a small room with a long table in front. At the table, men and women representing the gas drilling company sit. Some appear calm while others look down or away from the camera. The audience is respectful, but there is no respect for what the drilling company has done to this neighborhood. Off camera, a man states his name and address then asks, "What is the odor coming from the seven wells? It's unbearable. It's a terrible acrid odor. I have never smelled anything like that before. Is this going to be continuous, or what?"

The drilling company PR man answers that the impoundment initially held only freshwater but now it was being used to hold "flowback [waste] water," and that's why it's smelly. He says that the flowback consists of hydrocarbons, brine, and bacteria and that "the warmer it gets, the more putrid it gets." He promises that the drilling company will remove all the wastewater, replace the liner, and refill the impoundment with fresh water for now . . .

The man interrupts to ask if the odor will ever come back, and the PR man answers cautiously, "It may." The man then adds that sometimes he can't keep his windows open. Others in the audience agree, and then he asks if the smell is dangerous or harmful, and what are the hydrocarbons? Many people from the audience start shouting similar questions at the PR man all at once. He defers to a colleague, but the meeting is out of order and is temporarily halted to repeat the rules (standing up and stating names and addresses before each question).

The meeting resumes, with perhaps the most important questions left unanswered.

An elderly woman stands, gives her name and spits her words at the PR man. "I know you know who I am. I live right next to those wells, and that frack pit [wastewater impoundment] was put directly behind my home. You people have ruined my life. Wednesday night I had to call the emergency response system because we could not breathe up there. I am not going to tolerate this going on. You have ruined my property. I smell these smells all year long—it's not just a one-time thing because the weather got warm. I'm tired of all these people being all around my house twenty-four hours a day, lights on. I have no privacy, I don't even know who these people are around my house, and I'm there by myself now."

The PR man tries to calm her, for she is on the brink of breaking down. "It must have been hellish for you—"

She cuts him off hysterically. "That's an understatement! You almost gave me a heart attack when you flared that well. Do you realize what kind of hell you put me through? I don't think you do, I really don't think you do."

"We are working towards fixing that site," the PR man responds. "We plan to put screening up, trees—we are working towards undoing what we did." But his words, meant to calm, only inflame.

"What about the hell you put me through the last two years?" the woman demanded. "I mean, you don't have any idea! When they were drilling, the walls in my house were vibrating. And all this while my husband was dying—and it just went on." She breaks down sobbing, but collects herself to look at him one more time before sitting down and saying, "I'm done."

The PR man wisely does not respond to this woman, instead calling on a short, stout gentleman in the front row. This man sweeps his arm from one side of the table to the other and says that the drilling is happening across from his house, and now his property is "not worth nothin', can't give it away." He tells the men and women in the front about the structural damage on his house—damage caused by vibrations when the company put the road in. He has waited two weeks for a response from this drilling company and is now threatening to turn the matter over to his homeowners insurance, where it will be "Goliath against Goliath, not David [points to himself] against Goliath [points to the men and women at the front]." The PR man takes his number and promises to call.

There is a break in the recording; it continues with the PR man stating that the drilling company is looking at solutions, and if it means moving the impoundment, then that is what they will do. A voice, sounding like the elderly woman who spoke earlier, begs, "I just want you to move it, and get it away from my house." The PR man answers that it's not easy to move something that big, but agrees that yes, they'll take it away, but only if it's in everyone's best interest.

One clean-shaven middle-aged man stands up and states his name, and for a moment, it almost seems as if perhaps he will be the one who believes this drilling company really is a good neighbor, for he is speaking calmly. But it is not to be. He berates the men and women at the front for being poor neighbors since they first came into his community two years ago to clear the land. "You brought all these people in, did all this work, and never talked to a single homeowner about what was going on. You were in such a hurry to get that well punched in there that you didn't take time to talk to any of us." As he continues in a calm voice, the people in the audience turn to look at him, as do the company representatives sitting at the table. "Secondly," the man says, "none of you people have a stake in our community—none of you live here. We do. I'm here 24/7, I pay taxes, and I'm the guy that has to put up with this well site. The guy that owns the rights to that well site—he's not even a stakeholder in this community. Where they put the compressor station—that landowner is not a stakeholder in our community. None of these guys are stakeholders in this community. They don't live here. I do."

The PR man does not attempt to address these issues. No one interrupts. The man then continues, calmly, and now it seems that he has everyone's attention. "I plan to stay here. I got two little girls and a family. I think it's terrible what you guys have done. My property line butts right up to that well site. And you guys have wrecked my house. You guys have wrecked my community. You guys have come in here and made this a nonlivable community. You're like a family member who comes to visit and never leaves." He finishes forcefully, telling the men and women at the front, "Get done, and get the hell out." The room erupts in applause. In response, the PR man assures these people that what has happened in this community is an anomaly—is atypical for his drilling company. He then admits that this particular well site and impoundment were a disaster. It just didn't turn out the way they planned, that's all.

Even though the gas drilling company continued to assert that its operations had no impact on either family's water quality, Josie's and Sarah's water woes and their reluctance to keep quiet had by now gained the attention of the federal government. In July 2011, the EPA included Josie and Sarah in its study on the impacts of unconventional drilling on groundwater quality and tested their water as a part of that study. The EPA also invited two gas drilling companies to test both households' water at the same time: the company that was currently drilling on Mr. Leverkuhn's land and had previously arranged for Josie's and Sarah's water testing in November 2010, and a different drilling company.

The results from the drilling companies became available in the fall of 2011 (the results from the EPA would not become available until December 2012). Although one company initially withheld some of the data, the results of the testing done by the two companies eventually confirmed contamination of Josie's and Sarah's water sources. Especially concerning to me, as a mother and a veterinarian, was that three new chemicals ending in -*ene* were detected in their water: 2-methylnaphthalene, phenanthrene, and fluoranthene. Each of these three compounds belongs to a group of chemicals known as polycyclic aromatic hydrocarbons (PAHs), so named because they are composed of more than one fused aromatic ring (benzene has one aromatic ring). Because PAHs tend to persist in the environment and are easily absorbed, they have great potential to cause toxic or carcinogenic effects, or both. These are the chemicals that have been found to negatively impact fetal growth and childhood cognitive development.[23] These are also the chemicals that the FDA looks for in our seafood following oil spills, such as the Deepwater Horizon in 2010.[24]

As if being PAHs weren't enough, the 2-methylnaphthalene, phenathrene, and fluoranthene found in Josie's and Sarah's water also had another distinction: all have been identified as components of fracturing fluid and wastewater.[25]

After all the testing done on their water sources, no one informed either Josie or Sarah that her water was contaminated. More importantly, no one warned these families not to drink their water. Two years had passed since drilling operations began in their neighborhood, two years since they lost their water quality, two years since they lost their health and that of their animals, and yet no one was taking responsibility. No one was being held accountable. Another year would go by before they received advice, and even then, it would be muted.

The EPA tested Sarah's and Josie's water in July 2011 and March 2012. The cover letters accompanying the results stated that while the testing done on each woman's well water covered a broad spectrum of constituents, none were detected above the EPA's national primary and secondary drinking-water standards, except for nitrate and aluminum in Josie's water, and iron and manganese in Sarah's water. There was no warning *not* to drink the water, so did this mean their water was safe to drink?

It did not. But the families would not know this until later, when conference calls were held with EPA/ATSDR (Agency for Toxic Substances and Disease Registry) representatives to discuss the results of the tests and the potential health problems from continued exposure to each contaminant detected in the water. One simple question Josie and Sarah asked, one they'd been asking themselves all along, was, "Is our water drinkable?" The answer was "No. Your water is not drinkable. Your water is not potable."

Finally, someone confirmed what Josie and Sarah had suspected all along, but only verbally. Curiously, the EPA and ATSDR, for whatever reason, have thus far failed to put this advice to these families in writing.

When I first studied the EPA results, the last column, "MCL*" (primary maximum contaminant level), caught my eye, for most of the spaces in this column were blank. The primary MCL is the highest level of a contaminant allowable in drinking water;[26] without a primary

MCL, we don't know what the possible health effects or risks could be or will be. For example, in Sarah's EPA results, three semivolatile organics (2-butoxyethanol, phenol, and butyl benzyl phthalate) and one acid (formate) were detected in her water, and none of these has a primary MCL. The chemical 2-butoxyethanol was of particular concern. Used as a surfactant (foaming agent) in many fracturing fluid products, it is rapidly absorbed by all the major routes of exposure, including ingestion, inhalation, and through the skin. It can affect our red blood cells, bone marrow, liver and spleen,[27] and there is some evidence that 2-butoxyethanol could be carcinogenic.[28]

There was another problem with the MCLs, one voiced at several meetings I'd attended, including a recent Centers for Disease Control (CDC) conference on the health impacts of shale gas drilling. Because MCLs are set for exposures to individual chemicals only and not combinations of chemicals, we don't know the health effects of exposure to multiple toxicants, such as what Josie's and Sarah's families faced on a daily basis, possibly for months on end. Without knowing the primary MCLs of the contaminants in Josie's and Sarah's well water, no one can accurately predict the health problems they might face in the coming months and years, and no one was offering definitive answers.

In the spring of 2012, Sarah informed me that she and Josie were in litigation against all the companies and individuals involved in gas drilling operations and environmental testing associated with Mr. Leverkuhn's site. Pushed beyond the limit of tolerance, the women were fighting for their families' health, their animals' health, and their right to clean air and water.

Josie still awaits resolution of the civil proceeding against the PADEP. The drilling company, while not taking responsibility for changes in her water sources, has provided Josie's family with a water buffalo—twenty-five hundred gallons every five days since October 2011—something that is, according to Josie, very expensive. And while this helps, the water in the buffalo is not for drinking, and Josie and Jeff must continue to supply themselves with bottled water. Her family still suffers from headaches, nosebleeds, extreme fatigue, and a metallic taste in their mouths; the symptoms are exacerbated when flaring is taking place and the air becomes noticeably dense and smoky. In the spring of 2012, the family members were forced to leave their home for forty-eight hours when the air quality became intolerable, causing the people and the animals to gag and gasp for air. Josie's family developed large patches of raw blisters on the face, nose, and throat; the photos Josie showed me from this event look like people who have suffered chemical burns.

In the summer of 2012, Josie was blessed with a normal litter of puppies, the first in two years—no stillbirths, no malformations. Yet, the family is looking for property in states with no shale plays and with the acreage needed for their horses and dogs. "A hydrogeologist told us that what's in the water can be there for twenty to fifty years," Josie said. "That's a long time. What's our property going to be worth? Will they continue to give us water? We don't know the answers. Now, it's the air—we don't even know what we're breathing."

When I asked Josie what advice she could give people who are considering leasing their land, she gave these words of warning:

> I just want people to be aware. They [the drilling companies] paint such a pretty picture: there will be a little spot; they won't interrupt your life. But that's all it is—a pretty picture. They don't tell you about the traffic. They don't tell you about the hazardous chemicals you're exposed to. None of that money is worth it. Farmers are hardworking people. They want their lives easy. With fuel the way it is, with prices the way they are—they want an easier life too. You can't blame farmers for trying to take the easier way, especially when they [the drilling companies] paint the pretty picture. If people don't come forward and say things, people won't know that it's not a pretty picture. So they can say we're the crazy ones, but they'll see: they're not exempt from it.

As mentioned previously, Sarah and her children left their home for good after moving back in for only about a week at the end of the summer of 2011. They then stayed in Sarah's unheated camper until the end of the year, when the cold forced them to live with relatives and friends for months while they searched nearby for a home that would be big enough to accommodate all their animals. But most importantly, Sarah said at this time, "I just want a place to live and my kids to be healthy."

In June 2012, Sarah's family finally found a house to rent. She and the children began to recover their health here, and their animals' health improved, too; the cats lived with the family, but all the remaining animals—a horse, a donkey, a dog, and rabbits—lived with friends and relatives. Sarah's family felt settled for the first time in many months, but in May 2013 was forced to move again to another rental property.

As compressor stations and well pads continue to blot the landscape, Sarah realizes that any move is a gamble. At the end of a recent tour of her neighborhood, she pointed to a hill—fifty acres—owned by a friend who was approached by a company to lease the land for a compressor station. He knew everything that David had gone through, and Sarah warned her friend that it wasn't worth it: "If you want to ruin your family, your kids' and all your neighbors' lives, then go right ahead."

According to Sarah, the compressor station was never built, because people living beside the fifty acres refused to allow pipelines to cross their property. "They were worried about health problems," Sarah said. "They knew everything we went through."

In August 2013, Sarah decided to buy the second rental home, even though it wasn't large enough for all the animals and she hadn't sold her first home yet. The family was tired of moving, she told me, and I could hear the weariness in her voice, born of fighting for her family's health and her home for too many years.

Once more, I dare to hope that things will begin to turn around for this family. But Sarah's faith in her ability to survive this ordeal was tested again soon after she purchased the new home. During a routine check of her family's first home, she found that the doors had been ripped off, the wood burner and air conditioner stolen, copper piping and sinks ripped out of the walls. Police and insurance investigators' questions kept her too long at this house—where she seems to become ill more quickly with each visit—and after more than three hours, she was sicker than she has been in a long time, with stomachache, headache, a metallic taste in her mouth, and burning in her nose and throat. These things will clear up soon if she stays away, she told me, but the rash on her face has returned with a vengeance, and this will take a long time to resolve.

More than four years have passed since Sarah and Josie's neighborhood was invaded. Both women dream of selling their properties, but who will buy homes with tainted water and air and located in a neighborhood surrounded by well pads, compressor stations, and impoundments? Who will buy a home that has been vandalized because it has been sitting too long and subsequently lost its homeowners' insurance (as Sarah's did)? As more wells are drilled, more neighbors are experiencing the impacts that Sarah and Josie have described: the noise, the smell, the changes in the water, the health problems. And during that time, other neighborhoods have been invaded. More water buffaloes have appeared outside homes. More people spend as much time as possible away from their neighborhoods, and when home, stay inside with the windows shut. More community meetings are being held, more people shout and sob, and more representatives from the drilling company sit at the front of the room, wring their hands, look away, and deny responsibility for any problems.

Many proponents of gas drilling consider families such as these sacrificial lambs. They have lost their way of life so that the rest of us can continue to enjoy ours. We can purchase our 100,000-BTU barbeque grills and heat our poorly insulated homes to seventy-five degrees in the dead of winter. They are told that they are being patriotic, supplying the energy needs to our country so that we do not have to import oil from the Middle East. At the same time, multinational corporations are purchasing leases in Pennsylvania and planning to ship the gas to China and other lucrative markets. In most cultures, lambs that are sacrificed are treated with some respect, objects of reverence before the ultimate deed. Our sacrificial lambs are objects of derision that are cast aside and made to beg for water.

. . .

And what of the farmer, Mr. Leverkuhn, who unwittingly started this downward spiral for these two families and the entire neighborhood? On a tour of gas drilling development in her community in August 2012, Josie slowed down just after leaving her driveway and pointed to a steep dirt road on the right, leading up to the Leverkuhn well pad and impoundment. On the left side of the access road, there was recent excavation—remodeling of the site, according to Josie. I had been hearing about this pad, the wells, and the impoundment for over eighteen months, and now I desperately wanted to see it—this place that had brought so much grief to these families. But there was a sign at the entrance forbidding trespass, and Josie warned, "There are guards here 24/7." A little further on, Josie motioned to a spot where a new water well was recently dug, apparently because Mr. Leverkuhn had lost all his water. But now, there was talk of drilling another water well for Mr. Leverkuhn "clear up on that hillside, away from everything," she said, gesturing broadly to a rise in the distance. "Away from where the water is contaminated."

According to Sarah and Josie, Mr. Leverkuhn is being provided with bottled water and a water buffalo for his family and his beef cattle. They say he is embarrassed by this turn of events, that he is a proud farmer but hides the water buffalo behind a small hill, out of the neighbors' view, and continues to send his cattle to slaughter.

Mr. Leverkuhn did not return my calls.

THREE

SAMANTHA AND JESSE
Shattered Dreams

Livelihood: a means of support; subsistence. This word came up frequently during my conversation with Samantha Waller. It's how she got started breeding Newfoundlands, and it's why health—that of her and her partner, as well as her bitches, puppies, and studs—is such a complex issue. It's the reason her neighbor sold his cattle, bought a dump truck, and is working for the drilling industry. And it's why, after six years of breeding dogs, she has a full-time job outside the home because she and her partner are down to just a few dogs, and breeding is all but impossible anymore.

Bradford County, Pennsylvania, is, first and foremost, a rural, farming area. Leaving the main road in my small Prius was a challenge—with deep ruts and boulders everywhere, the roads were built for pickup trucks. But country roads have been a fact of life in Bradford County for decades. What has changed in recent years is the traffic on the main roads. Traveling through Towanda, the county seat (population about three thousand), can take as long as traveling across New York City in rush hour. Drilling traffic is nonstop, and lines of trucks bring traffic to a standstill seemingly for hours. This is the center of the gas drilling boom in northeastern Pennsylvania. Drilling permits are in place for a full build-out of the county—a process that will eventually extract gas from the Marcellus Shale in every corner and hamlet. But only a small fraction of the planned wells have been drilled, many have not been hydraulically fractured, and most of them are not yet producing. Nevertheless, traffic was incessant, and my attempt to get to where I was going was an exercise in frustration.

As I pulled into Samantha Waller and Jesse Klein's driveway, I didn't notice the dogs at first. I fumbled for notebooks and cameras and momentarily forgot that Samantha and Jesse bred Newfoundlands. Still and quiet, they were watching me, waiting for me to make the first move. Samantha greeted me just as I noticed her stoic giants, patient behind a pasture gate, calm and politely curious even after Samantha quickly introduced me to each of the half dozen dogs that were lounging in her large yard. The kennel was next door, and Samantha promised a complete tour and more time with her dogs after the interview.

Samantha is tall and has a commanding presence, a broad smile, and a deeply resonating voice. A self-proclaimed country girl from a family where music and farming are important, she moved from Bradford County to the outskirts of Philadelphia straight out of high school and played with her band that still includes a brother on the sound board. After ten years in the city, she missed the peace and quiet of the countryside.

"I moved here because I grew up here and I went to school here," she said, "and it's just the country and the fresh air. I can tell you the difference when I moved here from the Philadelphia area—I could breathe again."

Three years before unconventional gas drilling hit her neighborhood, she returned to start a dog-breeding business and a farm with her partner, Jesse.

"Before, you'd be lucky if you passed two cars and an Amish buggy on a fifteen-minute drive into town," Samantha said. "Now, I can't even get down to Leroy before I'm sitting in traffic behind hordes of water trucks and dump trucks, or big trucks that have huge things on 'em that take forever to drive down the highway. When these trucks are sitting in a line, all you smell in the valley is diesel fuel. Before, all you had to worry about was the odor of cow poop. Before, you could go outside at night, shut your eyes, and listen to the crickets, the peepers, and maybe hear a coyote howl. Now, if you go out my front door at night, all you hear is, beep, beep, beep and boom, boom, boom!" she said, clapping her hands loudly.

It's the sound of trucks backing up, crews building pads, drilling holes to preserve leases, and then moving on to build the next pad and lock the next lease. Without activity, the lease could be lost. And many leases were up for renewal in this neighborhood.

Samantha and Jesse's situation is not uncommon—they own the surface rights, but a local farmer, who sold them the house and the land, owns the mineral rights, which he leased to a gas drilling company. The farmer recently passed away, and the rights and the lease now belong to his spouse and children. "We didn't know what was going on until they [the drillers] were here," Samantha said. "Everyone was excited at first, thinking about how much money they were going to make. They didn't think what could happen. And now everybody is like, 'Ah, this is crazy! I can't sleep, I can't get to town.' Many people say it feels like we're being invaded. Aliens. They're everywhere. No matter where you go. And that's a sad, sad thing, because how do I know they won't come on our property?"

Samantha and Jesse's ten acres are situated on the corner of two narrow dirt roads on the side of a mountain just a short distance to downtown Leroy and nearby Canton. Next to their gravel driveway, a sign advertises brown eggs for a dollar a dozen. Samantha and Jesse's Rhode Island Red chickens live in a coop out back and share space with Piglet, the potbellied pig. The Newfoundlands' kennel is up front, right next to the driveway. On the other side of the driveway is their garden, in raised beds. The front porch looks down into the valley and across to the other side. From here, it's not obvious that within ten miles of this property, there are approximately four hundred permitted gas wells, most of these high-volume, hydraulically fractured Marcellus wells.

On a tour of Samantha and Jesse's neighborhood, we passed many unkempt properties with grass overgrown and appearing to be abandoned. Samantha pointed to three houses, part of what used to be a working farm. "This guy had a business," she said. "There were cows grazing here. This all happened in the last six months. People have been displaced from their homes, and the drillers have moved in. People who were renting—they can no longer afford to rent."

We drove onto a newly widened road that was once a one-laner, a back road used by teenagers to avoid the police after a night of heavy drinking. We passed many places where steep sides of hills rose twenty or so feet before flattening to a several-acre area, some topped by drilling rigs, condensate tanks, compressors, and trucks. Some appeared to have nothing on top, while many had grayish vegetation leading down one corner of the outside slope—places where chemical spills probably occurred or where wastewater may have run off the pad. Some of these flat areas appeared wet, others dry. Many had cornfields below them, and all were surrounded by either grazing deer or cattle, or sometimes both.

Samantha promised that we would see a lot today because "every back road leads to a well or well-related activity." Just a few minutes from her home, we stopped near one of the pads. Although we couldn't see very much, we could hear the sound of many trucks going by and compressors running. "This is the one closest to me," Samantha explained. "There was a spill of 420 gallons of concentrated hydrochloric acid and several thousand gallons of wastewater at this well site in 2009. It contaminated a pond and killed a thirty-foot swath of vegetation less than a mile from my home. Nobody was told. I didn't know. I didn't even know what 'frack' meant at that time. Now, I know when something happens. I'll see fifty white pickup trucks flying by, blinkers on." The water from the spill was never tested, and although the acid was neutralized, some of it undoubtedly leaked into the bedrock.[1]

I wanted to drive up closer so that I could get some pictures. "Oh, they won't let you—they'll arrest us!" Samantha said, pointing to the signs on the billboard at the entrance to the pad. In addition to the large No Trespassing sign, another sign read:

$ CASH REWARDS PAID $
For information leading
to the arrest and/or conviction
of anyone committing
a crime on this location.
ENERGY CRIME STOPPERS
888-645-TIPS

And in small print at the bottom, this curious sign assured anonymity.

After giving this sign careful thought, I felt empowered to call the number listed and collect my reward. This land is being violated both above and below the ground. I could report the name of the drilling company (easy enough—it's on the sign) and say what the land looks like and what the air smells like in this particular spot. I could join the ranks of energy crime stoppers in several other states including Texas, and remain anonymous!

We drove on, and Samantha asked me to stop again. "Now you can see where the runoff is," she said. "Those big black things are supposed to stop a leak from going down to the creek." She was referring to the booms, what we had seen on this tour at the base of all the pads and impoundments. Some booms looked like big black tubes, and others were substantial tubular cushions held in place by posts. We continued on a little further, following a boom as it snaked along, and we observed many areas where the runoff had sneaked past the boom, making its way effortlessly into the ditch at the side of the road.

Soon we reached the site of one of the best-publicized gas drilling spills in Pennsylvania, where thousands of gallons of flowback blew out during an initial stage of hydraulic fracturing, flooding the well pad before surging into a cow pasture, a tributary, and, finally, Towanda Creek. Six months later, beef cows grazed lazily below the pad, as if nothing had ever occurred here. The sides of the pad facing the road were very white, like they were covered with snow. I was glad to see that a fence separated this herd from the white-sided slope, but as the pasture lay directly below the pad, I wondered if anyone was monitoring the soil, grass, and surface water for contaminants from the slope runoff, contaminants such as the heavy metals, minerals, and radioactivity that were found to be elevated in nearby water wells following the blowout,[2] contaminants that would tend to stay in the soil, be absorbed by the grass, then eaten by the cattle in this pasture. I wondered if the steak and hamburger made from this herd would contain these contaminants.

And what about the cattle, including pregnant cows and calves, that were on this pasture at the time of the blowout—what exactly had they been exposed to? Later I learned that the company had released the names of some of the chemicals used in the hydraulic fracturing process on the FracFocus website, but only after repeated calls from the news media. In a case like this—an emergency situation where families were evacuated—all chemicals used should have been disclosed to the public and to health-care providers immediately after the accident, if not before.

Leaving this well site, we passed many pads and impoundments. At several sites, the cows stood in the barn or huddled just outside while trucks rumbled in and out, transporting gravel, building the pads. The cows appeared on edge, vigilant. On sites where bulldozers were breaking ground, bright orange flags were strung across the entranceway, giving the construction a festive appearance. Samantha called these "grand-opening flags." They were ubiquitous.

As we headed back to her house, I asked Samantha if I could ask her neighbors a few questions.

She shook her head and frowned. "No!" she replied. "They are too afraid to talk. You start talking about things like I did in the last couple months, and all of a sudden, every hour, you got white trucks going slow by your house."

I was surprised and asked for specifics.

"We had one [truck] the other night," she said. "They were going so slow, and staring at us. Jesse was on the front porch and said, 'What is this guy doing?' And so I went out, and we stood there and watched 'em. It was four guys with cowboy hats, just gave us the eye while they drove by real slow. A lot of people be scared by that."

Returning to Samantha's house, we passed several gas wells sitting on a pad above a veal calf barn, with rows of corn growing just beneath them. Samantha described what had been on her mind as well as the minds of other farmers.

"There are things that people don't think about when they're driving through here. People aren't thinking, 'Hmmm. We just passed a table of fresh fruits and vegetables for sale.' Or like at our house—farm-fresh eggs for sale. I want to know, how fresh are these things when there is a wastewater pond or hydraulic fracturing going on just a hundred feet away from where the vegetables were grown? How good will the fish from Towanda Creek taste after all that wastewater flowed into it following the Leroy blowout? How about the field corn that grows where runoff has occurred? Nobody is thinking about how that corn will be fed to cows or pigs."

I was hoping, at least, that the fields where sweet corn is grown were nowhere near any well pads. But Samantha drew my attention to fields of corn surrounding a well pad we were passing. "All that corn you see is sweet corn that's sold at produce stands and markets all around here."

We were nearly back to her place, yet we continued to pass pads. I ran a quick tally in my head—we had passed nearly twenty pads and had been on only two roads.

"Leaves you speechless, doesn't it?" Samantha asked. "And there are thirty pads on the other side of the valley I could have shown you."

I remembered what Samantha had said when we started out and how I found it difficult to believe—every back road leads to a well or well-related activity. Finally, we were on the road that led to her house—a road also not exempt, as she and Jesse have lately observed trucks driving by, loaded with drilling equipment. They suspect it is for construction of the well pad that will soon sit behind their home.

"I'll know when the grand-opening flags go up," Samantha said. "I'll be standing out there with my shotgun, saying, 'Don't you bend a blade of grass!'"

Several adult Newfoundlands sat behind the gate that opened to the backyard and kennel. As I greeted them, they gently wagged tails and heaved their heft to meet me eye to eye. Samantha reintroduced me to each of the eight dogs, showed off her pristine kennel space, and then filled up a black five-gallon bucket with water. It bubbled for a few seconds before turning pearly white, looking like 7-UP with milk added to it. After a few minutes, the water began to slowly clear. Later, in the house, she held a glass for me to sniff—it smelled like a sewer and caused my handheld methane detector to buzz like a beehive. According to Samantha and Jesse, the water doesn't always smell like a sewer—some days it smells like turpentine. And some days, it will have black or brown specks, or sand. And yes, they say, they can light their water on fire.

Ever since they have lived at this location, Samantha and Jesse have bought bottled water for themselves when they could afford it, because they don't like the taste of the well water either before or after it has gone through the water softener. But the dogs never seemed to mind the well water and in fact thrived on it. When the water quality changed in the summer of 2009, Samantha wrote it off as caused by the drought that year. It wasn't until the end of 2009 that she suspected that something was seriously wrong with her water.

"We started to have all kinds of issues with our animals," Samantha said. "We lost about seven chickens suddenly—we found them dead on the floor of the coop in the morning after looking fine the day before. And we started having trouble with the dogs—they wouldn't drink the water, and they began to have problems getting pregnant."

When I first heard about Samantha's dog-breeding problems in the summer of 2011, I suggested she get the dogs off the well water. Samantha reminded me of this now, two months later, as we talked at her kitchen table. Her Newfies, at 150 pounds each, are big drinkers— about a gallon of water per dog every day—and that's not counting the extra water needed in the summertime, to cool off and for bathing. Even though these dogs are Samantha and Jesse's livelihood, the women can't afford to provide the dogs with bottled water. So they began to catch and save rainwater. But this wasn't enough, so all of their animals, including the dogs, were forced to drink the well water.

In the spring of 2010, Samantha and Jesse began hauling water from a friend's well to supplement their water—for drinking and cooking, and to provide some freshwater for their dogs, cats, chickens, and pig. In 2011, they began hauling much more water—forty to fifty gallons every three to four days. But in the wintertime, the hauling was tougher because they used an outside hose to fill up their gallon jugs and went without when temperatures stayed below freezing. I wondered if they had complained to the PADEP and to the drilling company. In similar cases, bottled water is sometimes supplied for drinking, and a water buffalo is provided for all other water usage such as bathing, laundry, toilet flushing, and dishwashing. Yes, they did complain, but they were not provided with a clean water source.

Samantha and Jesse's well water was first tested in June 2011, as a "complimentary" test from the drilling company; a predrill test was never conducted. This test and later tests done by both the drilling company and the PADEP demonstrated high methane levels as well as levels of arsenic, manganese, and iron above the maximum contaminant levels. But because there were no predrilling tests on these substances, it's hard to say if drilling was the cause of these elevated levels in their well water. However, it is unlikely that methane levels were this high before drilling began. Before drilling started, Jesse never had a cucumber blown out of her hand while cleaning it under the faucet, and their water didn't look like fizzy milk, which in drilling areas is often due to the presence of fine methane bubbles. According to recent research, the average methane level in water in nondrilling areas in Pennsylvania is 1.1 milligrams per liter.[3] According to a test the PADEP conducted in November 2011, methane levels of Samantha and Jesse's well water reached 14 milligrams per liter, which is above the level deemed to be safe by the US Department of the Interior.[4]

Samantha and Jesse moved to Bradford County with the dream of breeding Newfoundlands in the country, where the dogs would have fresh air and clean water, and plenty of space. But they also dreamed of becoming farmers: raising calves and chickens, growing their own crops, producing their own food, and making crafts for the local farmers' markets.

When they first arrived at their new home in 2006, they had several cats and three Newfoundland adults and one puppy. Soon after that, Samantha acquired Piglet. I quickly learned that Piglet has a fierce desire to be photographed and to preach to the choir. Although I must admit that I'm not sure what Piglet was trying to say, I did enjoy taking photographs of him. Piglet now shares his shed with some of the chickens that were purchased in 2007 and kept free-range for egg and meat production. In 2009, Samantha and Jessie purchased two bull calves and raised them for meat.

During 2007 and 2008, Samantha and Jesse were in heaven: they were establishing themselves as breeders of top-notch Newfoundlands, and they were making a serious go at being farmers—and enjoying it. They bought more dogs and had litters on schedule—their breeding was going well and all the animals were healthy. But they left nothing to chance. In addition to regular health checks on all the dogs and puppies, they stayed with the pairs during breeding, ensuring good locks—when the male and female are end to end, and mating occurs—and preventing injury by literally wrapping their arms around the dogs, holding them together for fifteen to twenty minutes. To stay with the dogs as they gave birth and to watch the puppies afterward, Samantha and Jesse converted their basement into a maternity ward and added a comfy couch, a TV, and a fridge, so they could be with their dogs 24-7.

Samantha explained that some breeders leave the pups with the bitch and walk away. "They're so large, it's almost like raising pigs. They may lie down on two puppies and not realize it. It's critical for the first seven days—we don't take our eyes off of them, because it's our livelihood. We pull the pups off mom, put them on a scale, make sure they're gaining weight, then put them back with mom, making sure they have a good suckle [reflex]."

In the summer of 2009, Caesar, the stud they had brought with them as a puppy from Philadelphia, failed to produce litters. Previously, all six of Caesar's breedings had resulted in successful litters. As they could not afford to have Caesar medically evaluated and tested, they continued to breed him, but finally gave up and had him neutered and adopted in June 2011. At this time, Livia, a four-year-old female that had produced normal litters up until this time, had two stillborn puppies out of a litter of six, and developed rashes on her chest and stomach, and ear infections, as did many of the other dogs. During the next two heats, she was bred but failed to become pregnant. Like Caesar, she had been one of the original breeders at the farm, and like Caesar, she was neutered and adopted.

Since then, six females and five studs—three of these five studs brought in from areas where no gas drilling has taken place—have had an unusual number of unsuccessful breeding attempts while at Samantha and Jesse's kennel. In many of these cases, the females suffered from pseudocyesis, also known as false pregnancy, a condition that is common in bitches that are not bred after a heat cycle. For Samantha and Jesse, it was like an epidemic of pseudocyesis. "They [the dogs] were breeding, they were locking, their bellies would actually swell up," Samantha recalled. "And when it'd come time, they'd dig, make a nest, and no puppies. These girls were even making milk. At one time, we had four adult dogs down there waiting to have puppies, and not one had a puppy."

However, some of the dogs continued to have puppies, and this made it especially hard to point a finger at which bitch or stud might have been having fertility problems. To complicate matters, on a few occasions, outside owners brought in their own bitches to mate with Samantha and Jesse's studs, and the females did not produce litters from these matings.

I asked Samantha about medical evaluation to determine the cause of infertility in the dogs with problems. Specifically, I wondered what some basic health screens, heavy metal screens, and hormonal assays might show. I wondered if endocrine disruptors might be one of the causes of her dogs' breeding problems. But to rule that out, we needed to know the exact chemicals that were used in drilling and hydraulic fracturing on the nearest wells, know which chemicals returned to the surface in the wastewater, and then test for them. I was hoping that Samantha and Jesse had done some basic testing on at least some of the dogs. "I wish I would have," Samantha explained. Because this is their business, their livelihood, she and Jesse have sacrificed a lot of energy and time for the dogs and have gone without so that the dogs and puppies could have their physical examinations and vaccinations. But with the onset of breeding problems, Samantha and Jesse's income dropped precipitously, making their budget unbearably tight and impossible for them to spend the kind of money it would take to search for answers.

Samantha was used to belting out classic rock at nightclubs in the area, but she had recently stopped because of a constant burning in her nose and throat, a hoarseness to her voice, and a laryngitis that refuses to go away. Now she's hoping that the break in singing will allow her voice time to recover. Jesse, who cleans houses in her spare time, has had problems with her teeth—they seem to be hardening, becoming brittle and breaking; the dentist advised bone grafts. And while she had migraines before moving here, they were now occurring more frequently and were more severe. But when she leaves town to clean houses in Grover, about twenty minutes away, she feels better. "When I get out of this air," she says, "my nose opens up. I can breathe. I don't feel blah, tired." Both women have had episodes of gastrointestinal cramping, vomiting, and diarrhea after drinking the water and cooking with it. Both women have suffered drastic weight loss. Slight and frail, Jesse lost approximately thirty pounds in the past twenty months, while Samantha lost over one hundred pounds during the same time. What is striking to Samantha is that she hasn't changed her diet—she still eats as she did before, but continues to drop pounds.

I asked if they had been to the doctor for their health problems. Because they don't have health insurance, they avoid going to doctors unless absolutely necessary. The dogs' health care, it seems, trumps theirs, for at least the dogs have yearly physicals and vaccines.

While we were talking, a white pickup truck drove by, and both Samantha and Jesse jumped up to get a better look. (For some reason that neither they nor I understand, drilling company workers often seem to drive white pickup trucks.) Because of the harassment that Samantha and Jesse had described previously, I certainly understand why they are vigilant whenever they see a white truck—they not only feel threatened but are also worried. They believe it may be the beginning of much more traffic to come as the drillers were building a bridge that would provide easy access to their road.

Although Newfies are known for their stoicism, I wondered how their dogs would handle the traffic and the workers. Both women said workers have driven by their place several times, stopped their white trucks, and taunted the dogs until they begin barking and fighting with each other. Samantha and Jesse have had to run out and chase the workers away. I was reminded of an experience I had in Bedford County, Pennsylvania, when I stopped to take some pictures of a storage well during another interview. A gas company worker, while illegally recording the conversation without my permission, had tried to stop me from taking photographs but explained in no uncertain terms what a good neighbor he was. After asking whether I was one of "them activists from New York," he went on his way. Perhaps he, as well as the workers in the white truck that Samantha described, have a different view of what a good neighbor should be.

I asked Samantha if she planned to stay here, breeding dogs.

"I'm terrified," she answered. "But do I continue? Do I spend another eight thousand dollars for dogs, bring 'em here, and make 'em sick? Do I do this, or do I just go to work for the gas company? This [dog breeding] has always been my dream. And I know of people who have moved away from a gas well, only to have a gas well put right next to them. So I don't think there's anywhere we can escape from this."

Before departing, I asked to see their free-range flock. Samantha led me around to the side and back of her house, through long swaths of grass. Her Rhode Island Reds spied us and came running full speed toward Samantha, like mini velociraptors, but stopped on seeing me. Instead, they detoured to the unpaved road that winds up toward the mountain behind their coop, and they began to dig at the dirt and roll in it. Under normal circumstances, dust-bathing is a healthy behavior, performed by chickens to keep the lice and scales on their skin to a minimum. But because this particular dirt road is periodically sprayed with drilling wastewater, apparently to keep the dust down, the act of dust-bathing may be more akin to taking a toxic-chemical shower.

Samantha called to her chickens, and several ventured up to say hello. "See the one closest to the road?" she asked. "Her feathers are missing." Not only were feathers missing, but from where I stood, the skin appeared red and inflamed. I noticed several other birds with similar featherless red patches. I looked at the dirt and grass along the side of the road: the dirt appeared clumped and hardened with a film on top, and the grass looked as if it had been misted with oil.

"They [the drillers] just did this yesterday. They're doing it 'complimentary,' to keep the dust down," Samantha said sarcastically. "We call it 'fracking down'—they're just fracking us. They're just spraying the frack water everywhere."

Apparently, the wastewater spreading has been happening for the past several months, starting in the summer of 2011, and the lesions on Samantha and Jesse's chickens began appearing approximately one month after the spreading began. Remarkably, when the wastewater was being spread on Samantha and Jesse's roads, the use of drilling wastewater as a dust suppressant was illegal in Pennsylvania. I informed Samantha of this, and she laughed before asking, "Who's gonna stop 'em?"

As we walk around the back of the house, I asked about soil tests: there were none done as yet, but it was on the to-do list. I also asked about air tests. At the time of my visit, no air testing had been done, but exactly one week later, Samantha and Jesse's air was tested. Among the chemicals detected were chloromethane, trichlorofluoromethane, 2-butanone, carbon tetrachloride, trichloroethene, and toluene. I have seen these same chemicals detected in air tests from other rural properties in intensively drilled areas in Pennsylvania. In all cases, there were no pre-drilling air tests done, making it difficult to know if gas drilling is the culprit. Yet, should we expect to find these chemicals in the countryside? Would they have been detected if the land wasn't morphing into a gas drilling industrial zone? For now, there are no easy answers.

The view from Samantha's backyard opens into a very large field ending at the forest's edge. Here, Samantha and Jesse's ten acres meet the neighbor's land. This is where a well pad will soon sit, the well pad that will be in their sight all the time, a well pad on their back road. When I asked, "What will you do when this well goes in?" I realized that I was putting myself in her place and asking, "What would I do?"

She reminded me that one neighbor had sold his herd of cattle and bought a dump truck to start hauling water for the drilling company. "I'm not going to work for them," she said. "There's no way I would work for them. The way I look at it, I could live here and be killed off long term, or go to work for 'em and die off quicker! They're not telling those guys up there on the pads hauling chemicals and getting frack water spilled on 'em the truth—they're not telling 'em that they're gonna get sick and die." I'm not sure if Samantha had read the CDC National Institute for Occupational Safety and Health study saying that oil and gas workers are seven times as likely to die on the job as workers in other industries,[5] but her understanding of these workers' health was dead-on (no pun intended).

I was thinking about her house, her dogs, her life, her options. She seemed able to read my mind. "I was sold my property with potable water, but now, if I were to put it on the market, would you buy it? Would you come here and buy this beautiful piece of property? If the water smells so bad, it makes you want to throw up? If you have to take a shower four hours before company arrives, so you can air the house out?"

She knew the answer to this question, but she was looking for advice—what should she do?

I had no clear-cut answers.

"I've spent forty years of my life to be able to get this, to be able to buy this property and farm this land, to have the American dream. And then corporations came in and took it away from us overnight."

In March 2012, Samantha started a full-time job in a gardening center, tending plants. At home, there are five adult Newfoundlands with uncertain futures. It's ironic that Samantha has found a job working in a gardening center, because she and Jesse had planned to have a greenhouse next year to produce veggies to sell at a small stand along with their farm-fresh eggs. Their goal for 2013 was to have thirteen breeding Newfoundlands along with the produce stand and a wood shop, but that seems impossible now. After repeated requests, the drilling company vented Samantha and Jesse's water well in April 2012. Since then, the women have noticed that the water spits and sputters less frequently, but they still occasionally see some sand and grit. According to Samantha, they continue to leave the door cracked open when they shower, just in case.

Driving away from Samantha and Jesse's home, I was reminded of the plans for Bradford and Tioga Counties. Looking at the map of leases and permits in these two Pennsylvania counties, it is clear that that the area will soon be saturated with gas wells. In fact, in all of Pennsylvania, only 2 percent of the projected number of wells have been drilled, and many fewer have yet to be hydraulically fractured.[6] You can drive around these counties, and except for the intense traffic and occasional industrial sites associated with gas drilling, the area remains beautiful and rural. But in this little area of the world, Samantha and Jesse's neighborhood, the build-out has begun. In their neighborhood, we can travel down roads with wells every few hundred yards, giving us an idea of what full build-out will look like.

The industry would like us to think that the industrialization of the area is just temporary and that everything will go back to normal after all the wells are drilled in ten or twenty years. But consider what is happening now in this small area that is being intensively drilled. In three years, there have been three major accidents within a three-mile radius. Two we have already discussed: the well that blew out during the hydraulic fracturing process and contaminated a tributary of the Susquehanna River and, a year later, the spill of 420 gallons of concentrated hydrochloric acid and drilling fluids. A third well was cited twice for a faulty casing.[7] Several months after the second incident, methane was still being detected in water wells and bubbling up in streams in the area.[8]

Is this what we have to look forward to for the next ten to twenty years? And after all the wells have been drilled, will life return to normal? The economic activity associated with the drilling will cease, and if the current production numbers are correct, the economic benefits from royalties will soon plummet. We will be left with tens to hundreds of thousands of holes in the ground where we have exchanged freshwater for toxic chemicals and hydrocarbons. These holes will be sealed with cement that will eventually fail, with unknown consequences for the drinking water of future generations.

FOUR

ANN AND ANDREW
Reluctant Refugees

The term *nostalgia* is often used to describe the emotional stress of homesickness. But when an environmental event changes your home or way of life, the longing for better times can produce a similar stress. The Australian philosopher Glenn Albrecht has coined the term *solastalgia*[1] to describe the distress caused by an environmental change directly connected to an individual's current home. In this way, the home can become an emotional prison, and the only solution is to leave and establish a home in a new environment. This is the story of a husband and wife who endured but recognized the perils of solastalgia at several locations. As this book is being written, they are considering yet another move.

When I first met Ann Smith and her husband, Andrew, in August 2012, they were living in their fourth residence. Over the past thirty-five years, they had moved three times to escape the health impacts of the fossil fuel industry, from nice homes sitting on nice pieces of property, to a beautiful home ten miles from their first house and surrounded by roads sprayed with drilling wastewater.

During our talk, both Ann and Andrew referred to their previous homes as *incidents*, as if their houses could be reduced to unpleasant events, rather than places where they had lived. It wasn't until we discussed their third move that I began to understand why. They told me about a neighbor who stayed on even though her health had been severely affected by the shale gas drilling in their neighborhood. When I asked why she didn't move, they explained, "She's lived there thirty-five years, and she'll never leave, no matter what."

"That's a hard thing for people to admit [that you must leave your home for the sake of your health]. I've gone through it with this one," Andrew said, pointing to a picture of Incident 3. "I said, 'I'm just gonna get the hell out of here. Move on.'"

Solastalgia, I thought. It's probably something you can never fully understand until experiencing it, and I hoped I never would.

About an hour south of Ann and Andrew's current residence, I observed miniature oil rigs on lawns, where geese or deer statues might otherwise have been. Very soon, I understood why. I was passing through Titusville, Pennsylvania, where Edwin Drake ("Crazy Drake") of the Seneca Oil Company and William "Uncle Billy" Smith together drilled the first successful oil well. They hit oil on August 28, 1859, near present-day Oil Creek State Park, using a drill fashioned by Smith, who was a blacksmith, and a pine derrick that they had built together. The discovery set off an oil rush, the echoes of which have spread throughout the world. But the oil boom was first felt in Titusville, where the population grew fortyfold within six years and where eight refineries were built within the decade. I had not realized that Ann and Andrew lived so close to Titusville, as they hadn't mentioned this landmark when we discussed directions. Then again, passing through Titusville, I wondered if the average person would have any idea that the first oil well was drilled in Pennsylvania. I suspected that most people would say somewhere in the Middle East or maybe Texas. But certainly not in Pennsylvania.

With photos spread on their dining room table—documentation from the three previous incidents—the Smiths were ready and waiting for me. A middle-aged couple from this region of Pennsylvania, they balanced each other perfectly. Ann is a short, energetic, quick-witted housewife, a horse breeder, and a self-described go-to person. Andrew is a tall, calm, and thoughtful businessman, the owner of a successful sawmill who has been in the lumber industry all his life.

When she wasn't leaving the room to find more documents in her files, Ann stayed seated during the interview and Andrew stood beside her, occasionally elaborating on her statements whenever the opportunity arose. Some of the photos on the table—close-ups of bubbles frozen in pond ice and of bubbles percolating from wet ground in the pasture and the dirt driveway—I recognized from Incident 3, the residence I knew the most about. But today my goal was to start from the beginning, from the first house, and move forward to where they lived now. I was particularly curious about what happened at Incident 1, because I grew up in a small town in south Jersey, surrounded by three large oil and gas refineries, and never realized what clean air and fresh water was until I moved to upstate New York.

Ann showed me a photo of Incident 1. A colonial mansion, built in 1863, sits high above the town, with tall windows all around and columns in front, reminding me of a luxurious antebellum Southern plantation home. It was in this house that Ann and Andrew began their life together. Andrew explained that his family owned nine hundred acres of oilfield in the area and that this house sat on four hundred acres of unleased land adjacent to the oilfield, not too far from where we were now talking. The Smiths lived there from 1978 to 1988, in their spare time restoring the mansion, which had been built and owned by Andrew's great-great-grandfather. While living there, they developed a high-grade herd of registered beef cattle, bred and showed horses, and had several beloved English mastiffs as pets. And while living there, Ann became very ill.

Because the Smiths had documented the events carefully, and because they sought help from politicians, reporters, the PADEP, and special commissions, I was fortunate to have mounds of records and letters to piece together what had happened to them. In mid-1981, Ann began to experience bizarre allergic reactions to many substances, with severe episodes of sneezing and nosebleeds. Although she was seeing an allergist, her symptoms seemed to intensify. Over the Christmas holiday in 1983, she developed stage IV status asthmaticus (a sudden worsening of asthma symptoms that are not responsive to treatment), with more episodes occurring over the coming months. For Andrew, who rushed an air-starved Ann to the emergency room countless times, life devolved into spending evenings in the ER and working during the day.

That year, before Ann's attack of status asthmaticus, the Smiths had noticed changes in the air and water quality. Their well water would periodically turn brown with white specks, and there was often a smell of sewage or rotten eggs in the air, so intense that it would force them to leave their home and stay in a travel trailer graciously lent by a neighbor. During 1986, the Smiths observed a fine white powder in their home and on their vehicles, lawn, and trees, and they and their animals had frequent health problems. Ann and Andrew suffered from blisters, nausea, headaches, nosebleeds, and a burning sensation while breathing. Meanwhile, their cat, dogs, horses, and cattle had recurring respiratory and skin problems, including blisters and hair loss.

In December 1986, Ann and Andrew discovered that not only did their neighbors have similar symptoms, but a spill of liquid naphtha—produced during the distillation of crude oil—had occurred at the oil refinery storage facility located on a neighborhood tank farm. They would later learn that spent catalyst powder, a fine white powder used in petroleum refining processing, was being deposited here.[2]

When I inquired about legal issues, I quickly realized that both Ann and Andrew were still distraught about all that had happened with Incident 1 and the refinery, particularly their lawsuit, even though it happened nearly twenty-five years ago. Raising her voice a pitch or two, Ann described the many hours spent in law, medical, and chemistry libraries researching refineries, catalyst powder, and environmental lawsuits. When she was finished recounting this to me, Andrew gave his opinion loudly and firmly. In contrast to the calm, soft voice he had been using, he now spoke more forcefully as he explained that from this experience, they learned that a lawyer may all too often make more money defending the fossil fuel industry than prosecuting cases for private citizens, such as themselves.

Their first move was to Jamestown in Chautauqua County, New York (Incident 2). There, the Smiths rebuilt a dilapidated farmhouse and barn and lived there from 1988 to 2005, on 135 acres, continuing to keep both their beloved horses and dogs. During the next nine years, both Andrew's and Ann's health improved, and both were happy to breathe the air.

But Incident 2 was less than thirty minutes away from Incident 1 and the refinery. "Why not move further away?" I asked.

"There were two big positives," Andrew answered. "We were still near the business, and there was no hydrocarbon extraction in the area."

Yet. Although they moved when there was little drilling activity in the immediate area, this part of New York has been the most intensively drilled area for both oil and gas since the nineteenth century. In fact, William Hart drilled the first commercial gas well only thirty miles away from Incident 2 in Fredonia, Chautauqua County, in 1821. Hart, a local gunsmith, first dug a twenty-seven-foot-deep well and then drilled to seventy feet to reach a pocket of gas. He put in a gas meter and piped gas to a local innkeeper. In the next few years, Fredonia became known for gas-fired street lighting made possible by a multitude of shallow gas wells.

Today, while Chautauqua and Cattaraugus Counties in New York are not the largest producers of natural gas in the state, they do have the largest number of active gas wells. Although Chautauqua County is often noted as a place where tourism and hydrocarbon extraction and use can coexist, it remains the part of New York outside of the New York City metropolitan area with the poorest air quality. The Levant area of Chautauqua County is known for a 1980s case of gas migration to drinking water, which resulted in the explosion of a water well and contamination of a number of other water wells in the area. Gas wells had been drilled in the year prior to the explosion on a nearby hillside. Using radiocarbon dating, the New York State Department of Environmental Conservation (NYSDEC) showed that the source of the gas found in the water wells came from deep sources and was consistent with the gas produced from recently drilled gas wells.[3] So, while the Smiths moved at a time when drilling south of Incident 2 was not particularly active, the area was no stranger to hydrocarbon extraction.

The Smiths explained that when they bought Incident 2, they bought both the surface rights and the mineral rights but that a previous owner had leased these rights to a drilling company. Because their research indicated that no drilling was likely to occur, they thought they were safe, but they hadn't researched their neighbors' opinions on the subject. They soon discovered that almost everyone around them wanted gas wells, and in 1997, Ann and Andrew were introduced to the world of gas drilling. The first well, approximately nineteen hundred feet away, was conventional, using approximately sixty thousand gallons of water and chemicals. After the hydraulic fracturing was completed, the Smiths' water quality changed, slowly becoming too salty to drink and forcing them to buy bottled water and haul water for their horses. So the Smiths drilled another water well. "The first water well we had was at a hundred thirty-five feet," Andrew explained. "We went down ninety feet on the second well and had potable water. The crazy thing was, the neighbors still wanted drilling."

According to the Smiths, after the first gas well was drilled, their health and the health of their animals again began to decline. "We found out we really couldn't take the rock cuttings, neither one of us," Ann said. There was a period of approximately two years in between bursts of drilling. During drilling events at Incident 2, the Smiths experienced health issues similar to what they had encountered at Incident 1: difficulty breathing, burning throats, mouth blisters, rashes, upset digestive systems, and nosebleeds. "We'd take it for so many hours, but then we would get to the point where we couldn't take it anymore," Ann said. "We'd take off in the vehicles with our dogs for a few hours, detox, and come back. Often we'd sleep in our vehicles at Andrew's business."

But they couldn't take their horses, all coughing and heaving, and on steroids because of breathing problems. In 2003, the Smiths were evacuating every night because of the drilling, and it was hard to stay home during the day. At one point they vacated for a full month with all of their animals by leasing a barn for the horses and renting a travel trailer to stay nearby. Still, the horses may have suffered the most, because other than this month away, they rarely left the farm.

After the Smiths' experience with the refinery lawsuit at Incident 1, I truly doubted that they would have jumped into another fight with the industry. But they did. They were slow learners, Ann said, because over the next six years, they hired several law firms, most of which soon came to the Smiths asking to be released. The Smiths suspect that the lawyers were approached by the gas exploration company and promised large amounts of legal work. In their lawsuit, the Smiths asked basic questions about the fairness of land contracts and the rights to all water in a community. They asked moral and ethical questions. For example, does a drilling company owe a duty of care when operating in the vicinity of a heart or lung patient? If rock cuttings are considered hazardous waste if submerged in water, how can they be benign when blown indiscriminately into the air, especially if they can be inhaled?

"We took an unpopular stand, and we weren't very successful," Ann noted. "Our mission was not to prevent drilling; it was to force the exploration company to use diligence and care in the vicinity of a lung patient. We felt strongly that we should not be driven from our home."

Instead, according to the Smiths, 2005 arrived with a projection of more gas wells in their area. This, combined with soaring health insurance premiums due to a legal loophole between the two states, forced them to forsake the second place they had loved.

On the way to the Smiths' current home, I took a detour to the location of Incident 3, approximately an hour south from Incident 2, in Pittsfield, Pennsylvania. The property sat at the top of a very steep dead-end dirt road in the middle of thousands of acres of Allegheny Forest timberland. Just off the road were two ponds, and nearby, the farmhouse and barn sat on forty wooded acres spaced far from other houses, giving the appearance of complete privacy. I could understand why they fell in love with the place: it looked like a dream home.

The Smiths bought Incident 3 in 2005, remodeled the home, and rebuilt the barn, moving in 2006. They moved to escape the previous drilling company, but also because they were told the new area was not promising for hydrocarbon exploration. "We went to two different geologists from surrounding leaseholds, and they said 'No!'" Ann said, banging her fist on the table. "'No drilling in the foreseeable future. No drilling!'" She waved her arms in a complete circle, "Everything around us—dry!"

Andrew explained, "Even though we owned the surface and mineral rights, forty acres doesn't mean anything, because we were surrounded by others who had leased."

As they reminisced about moving into Incident 3 and their first years there, I noticed a distinct change in Ann's and Andrew's moods. "We had a blessed year and a half where things got really better. Air was wonderful, the water was clear and good. Horses got better. Dogs got better, we got better," Ann said calmly, as she and Andrew smiled at each other. "Ha! We were away from the drilling company, and I was able to get off my asthma medicine. The one mare that was having such respiratory problems, I was able to ride her, and we were thinking about showing her. We had plans—we were going to get on with our life. We rebuilt the barn and had a contractor lined up to rebuild the house, set back behind the ponds—something we felt we deserved."

In the summer of 2007, the PADEP called and informed the Smiths that a company was coming in to drill a vertical gas well within a mile of their home. "We couldn't get our minds or tongues wrapped around the word 'Marcellus'—it sounded so silly," Ann said, as if the word *Marcellus* tasted bitter. "We didn't have a computer, so I couldn't research this easily. We thought, they're just going to drill a test well, just one well. Then we were told four test wells—we had no clue what a test well was. Still, we thought, we could put our heads in the sand, we could evacuate, detox, come back. We could get through this."

"Forty-five hundred feet away," Andrew said. "We could tough this one out. And the prevailing winds would be away from us." Incident 3 was downhill from the well site, with a lot of woods to go through.

According to the well record and completion report supplied by the Smiths, drilling at this gas well lasted only five days in August 2007, and hydraulic fracturing took place twice over several days in August and October 2007. There is nothing on the record, however, about the venting that apparently occurred over the subsequent weeks. Soon after completion (hydraulic fracturing and production), the Smiths noticed that the air quality changed. They'd wake up in the middle of the night and feel as if they were suffocating. Andrew called the drilling company and the PADEP two or three times per week and complained that there was something wrong. He was told that there was nothing wrong with the new well site.

"So I began walking the hill where the gas well was," Andrew said. "And I found I couldn't breathe. I couldn't smell anything unusual; I just couldn't breathe."

The Smiths began evacuating on and off that fall of 2007, just as they had in their previous two homes. They managed to keep working and to keep their lives on track, but it took enormous energy and courage to do so. "I remember one night was so bad," Ann said, "I called the county fairgrounds and asked, 'If I have to evacuate these horses, can I bring 'em down?'" At this time, the Smiths discovered that an old gas pipeline, cutting across their backyard and close to the horse barn, was leaking. "The pipe had rusted through and the gas was bubbling into the pasture, sixty-five feet from the horse barn," Ann explained.

Christmastime 2007 is a time Ann and Andrew will never forget. There was a heavy snow that year, and Andrew had gone out to watch another pipeline repair on their property. On his way out, he was shocked to see that the large pond by the house was bubbling like a cauldron, with a hole through six inches of ice and two and a half feet of snow.

In the commotion to document this event, the Smiths found that both their and their neighbor's camcorders were dead. Ann and Andrew immediately called the drilling and pipeline companies as well as the PADEP. The next day, representatives from the drilling and pipeline companies arrived, but by then, the bubbling had stopped. The Smiths strongly suspected that under pressure, gas and flowback fluids had escaped onto their property through natural faults in the underlying rock.

In the coming months, both ponds bubbled and developed an oily sheen and white film, which Ann and Andrew also observed in their springhouse and well water. As they spoke, the Smiths showed me photos and videos of the ponds: bubbles in the winter caught frozen, and in the summer, an oily film with slick-coated bubbles. There are hours of footage with bubbles rising upward and breaking at the surface as if duck bubblers—aerators that keep duck ponds ice-free—had been installed.

The PADEP visited the Smiths' property many times after their pond's blow-out, sampling the water in their spring and pond, surveying the pond, and inspecting the gas wells closest to them. In September 2008, the Smiths received a letter from the agency stating that there was no indication that their waters were affected by oil- and gas-related activities.

In the end, neither the drilling company nor the pipeline company was held accountable. With arms crossed in front of her, fingers pointing in opposite directions, Ann said, "And the Smiths sat in the middle!"

.   .   .

From the stacks of letters and reams of test results and other records they kept, I can attest that the Smiths did more than simply sit in the middle: they were proactive in the strongest sense of the word. These were not people who needed encouragement to have testing done. The only thing they didn't do was to have a predrilling air test done—something that would have been extremely useful but expensive and often is difficult to perform and interpret. Without a predrilling test, one could spend thousands of dollars on air and water testing, as the Smiths had done for the third time, and have no chance to definitively point to any chemical or substance as the cause of the problem.

So why do it? What drove Ann and Andrew to go nearly bankrupt a third time in trying to find a cause through testing? The answer is simple: their own health and that of their animals. At Incident 3, the Smiths reported symptoms that were very similar to what they experienced in Incidents 1 and 2, with burning in the eyes, nose, and throat being the most common. They also noted additional problems: their skin felt like sandpaper, their teeth and jawbones ached, and they suffered from nausea, breathing difficulty, severe headaches, and heart-attack-like chest pains. Their horses and dogs suffered from multiple health problems, including respiratory difficulties such as severe wheezing and coughing that could only be lessened with large doses of steroids.

"After 2007, through 2008 and into 2009, things just got worse," Ann explained. "I really destabilized—I went back to being status asthmaticus. My sinuses got worse, my eardrums ruptured, I became deaf. Andrew and I suffered severe fatigue."

There's more, I thought, remembering the thick packet of lawyers' letters, names removed, that Ann had sent me months ago. Ann and Andrew were down for the third time. Why did they try again?

"If it gets to a point where we can't make headway, we do what we call Plan B, which is to pack up and move," Ann explained. But first they tried because they thought they had a fighting chance. "We took Incident 3 up to the point where I contacted five lawyers and finally retained one from Pittsburgh. I contacted twenty-one testing firms. A few of the really big ones were going to come in with air testing, were going to come in with water testing. The Pittsburgh lawyer told us we'd need three hundred thousand dollars to initiate and run the lawsuit, then we'd need another three hundred thousand if we got SLAPP suited [in a strategic lawsuit against public participation (SLAPP), a party is sued by the plaintiff in an attempt to stifle public criticism]. We just looked at each other and said, 'We can't live here. Period. So why don't we just move.'"

Still, they hesitated. In the early summer of 2009, the Smiths were notified that the drilling company was planning a second Marcellus well adjacent to the first. In light of their two-year nightmare, the Smiths asked the drilling company to buy them out, but their request was ignored. There was no other option but to secure a large mortgage, buy another house, and take another loss—this time over $500,000.

In the fall of 2008, during one of the many times the Smiths had evacuated Incident 3 to detoxify, they had passed through a neighborhood with many gas wells, within ten miles of Incident 2, and noticed an abandoned house and barn. By the summer of 2009, the property was theirs, and for the fourth time, they found themselves rebuilding a house and a barn. The house sat just off the road, on 75 acres with mineral and surface rights that were not leased, and was surrounded by several smaller unleased lots for sale, which the Smiths quickly bought, increasing their acreage to 115.

"What about the neighbors?" I asked, with trepidation.

"I went to the courthouse and looked up everybody's deed," Andrew said confidently. "Nobody around us is leased."

Ann added, "That was a big criterion. We're only here while there's a hiatus in drilling. We'll never be able to stand being next door—"

Andrew interrupted his wife. "We will not stick around," he said defiantly. "We know better than to try and fight. They have too much power."

Did they mean it? If drilling started near them, would they move yet again?

Ann answered calmly, "We take it day to day to day. You get up each morning, thinking, 'Is this the day I'll have to leave?' Because we wouldn't be able to stay. This time, if the drilling starts, it'll take me about five minutes to keel over."

I wondered whether they noticed a change in their animals' health after moving to their current location. Fortunately for the Smiths, most of the health problems their animals experienced at the previous location have abated. According to Ann as well as her farrier—who had spent the most time with the horses at Incidents 2 and 3 and continues to take care of the horses at the current location—the biggest change observed was in the horses' feet: they had improved dramatically since leaving Incident 3. And because it takes approximately a year for a horse to grow a new hoof, the horses' feet were continuing to improve. When I asked Ann if she was able to ride any of the horses yet, she smiled and answered in the affirmative that one particularly nice-looking horse often "hauled the royal 'ass' around the farm."

Regarding Ann's and Andrew's health, the answer was complex. Andrew no longer suffers from many of the acute respiratory, gastrointestinal, and neurologic symptoms that he once endured, but he still experiences the same extreme fatigue and weight gain that Ann did. Ann's hearing has returned, and her asthma is now stable. But since moving to her current home, she has developed imbalances in her parathyroid and adrenal glands, possibly due to the steroids taken for many years to control her asthma and sinusitis, although no definitive cause has been found. She doesn't blame any of these current health problems on this particular location, but does say that before Incident 1, she was as healthy as an ox. Photos taken at Incident 1, before she became ill there, show a woman who worked the farm; baled hay; drove a tractor; raised cattle, horses, and dogs; and took care of her home and man. According to Ann, years of exposure to endocrine-disrupting chemicals and years of medications to control her symptoms and keep her alive have taken a toll and her body is now worn out. At this location for more than three years, she is fighting hard to stay stable.

But where would the Smiths go? Would they stay in this area because of the business?

This time, it was Andrew who answered immediately: "No! I'll fold up at this point. I'll be sixty-two."

In September 2011, approximately two years after moving to their current residence, Ann sent a letter to the PADEP with photos detailing the dumping of drilling wastewater on nearby dirt roads. She is concerned that once the material is dried, the contaminants in the wastewater will be inhaled and will cover crops grown for animals and people. She worries about runoff into streams, marshes, and swamps. And she is concerned about rural water wells and the Amish children who often walk these roads. Months later, she sent me an update—the dumping continues, often in the wee hours of the morning, despite the No Brine signs in her township.

In early December 2012, just months after I first met the Smiths, Ann noticed an article in the newspaper announcing that liquefied natural gas export terminals would be built in the United States and that the immediate ramifications of this action would be increased exploration. Out of fear that drilling would drive them out yet again, she called a realtor and unofficially placed her home on the market.

Soon after, Andrew suffered two heart attacks within a week. Ann was worried about the business, although Andrew has told her to let the business die should he die. But luckily, he's still alive, and she's trying to learn it fast.

I remembered my talk with them a few months earlier, when I had asked about their plans and Ann had abruptly said that she would be dead in two years and she definitely expected to go first. Andrew had stood beside her, appearing strong and vibrant, and had laughed. "She's always saying that."

Andrew's massive heart attack, and then another three days later—this wasn't in Ann's plans.

Living in the shadow of Edwin Drake's oil well, moving from house to house, but never escaping the area, the Smiths have managed to survive financially but their health has been devastated. In the sense that they have let go of each home when the health consequences became overwhelming, they have overcome solastalgia. In another sense, however, northwestern Pennsylvania is their home and they have never left it, despite the consequences. As I write this, I think of this vibrant and fiercely intelligent couple with a wonderful sense of humor, looking at each other and trying to guess who will be the first to die before his or her time.

FIVE

FRACKING, FARMING, AND OUR FOOD SUPPLY

When you think of a typical farm, you might envision a small, idyllic couple of acres with several species of animals. But in reality, there's a range of farms, from tiny family plots to massive factory operations. Vast factory farms with economies of scale and modern farming techniques supply the majority of the food found in our supermarkets, but with significant environmental impacts.[1] In part because of health (e.g., the overuse of antibiotics and the use of bovine growth hormone) and environmental concerns about factory farming, smaller farms—particularly organic farms—are making a comeback. Nevertheless, what they all share is the need for clean water and clean air. And no matter the scale, consumers expect their food to be free from chemical contaminants and pathogenic organisms.

The production of food in the midst of unconventional drilling operations raises questions about the safety of food raised near such operations. As for food producers, the gas drilling boom in Pennsylvania has been promoted as a boon for farmers who lease their land and the savior of the family farm. Farms that had been going out of business can now buy new machinery, rebuild the barn, and pay off loans. However, some farms reluctantly go out of business because of gas drilling. Farming has been intertwined with the oil and gas industry in Pennsylvania for 150 years. Only in the last few years has gas drilling become increasingly profitable and increasingly disruptive. The strain that this gas industry expansion has put on food production and the associated issues of food safety are the themes of this chapter and chapters 6 and 7.

. . .

We have spent considerable time over the last few years with farmers: not large producers, but owners of relatively small family farms—those with the most to gain or lose from gas drilling. Making general statements about how farmers feel about this issue is impossible, as each farmer has his or her unique and sometimes colorful perspective. The only refrain that we have heard consistently is that farmers do not want to be told how to do their jobs or what they can or cannot do with their land. The main concern of these farmers is that gas drilling represents a landowner's rights issue. But even this leads to a range of opinions.

The issue of horizontal gas wells that use hydraulic fracturing has been dealt with very differently in Pennsylvania than in New York. In recent years, Pennsylvania has had a Republican-dominated legislature and a Republican governor, Tom Corbett, whose election campaigns have been supported by the generosity of the oil and gas industry. For the most part, laws have been passed that generally favor efficient extraction of oil and gas at the expense of the environment and health of the citizens of the commonwealth.[2] In March 2013, the PADEP agreed to have the nonprofit organization State Review of Oil and Natural Gas Environmental Regulations (STRONGER) review the department's regulatory program. STRONGER's September 2013 report indicated that the PADEP does in fact have regulations consistent with the standards expected by industry.[3] Little consideration was given to public health, food safety, or the implementation of the regulations.

In New York, the legislature is split between a Democratic-controlled Assembly and a Republican-controlled Senate, with a relatively conservative Democratic governor, Andrew Cuomo. For the last four years, New York has not permitted horizontal drilling with high-volume hydraulic fracturing, but has permitted most other forms of oil and gas extraction. Although by early 2014, the decision on whether to permit the use of unconventional oil and gas extraction in the state is awaiting a review by the New York State Department of Health, the regulations proposed by the state's Department of Environmental Conservation (NYSDEC) are among the worst in the country.[4]

Even though New York has not yet been touched by the shale gas boom, some people argue that when the rigs move in, farmers will finally get the money for their new barn and tractor, or maybe this will be the one thing that will save the family farm. The main concern of these farmers is that gas drilling represents a landowner's rights issue—"don't tell me how to use my land." Other farmers want nothing to do with drilling; they are worried about environmental degradation and do not want to lease their surface or mineral rights. They, like the farmers who embrace drilling, do not want anyone telling them what they may or may not do with their land, but if enough of their neighbors lease, they may be forced into a drilling unit against their will with minimal compensation. This is New York's compulsory integration law. This law (actually an amendment of Title 9 of Article 23 of the Environmental Conservation Law)[5] was written by Tom West (a lawyer with gas company clients),[6] sponsored by Republican senator George Winner,[7] and unanimously passed in the New York State Senate in June 2005. This was before shale gas extraction was on the radar of most New Yorkers (but very much on the mind of the oil and gas industry), and the compulsory integration law was thought to be a device to protect landowners.

Consider a conventional fossil fuel source such as a pool of oil or a pocket of gas, far beneath the surface but under both your property and your neighbor's. If your neighbor puts in a vertical well and sucks the gas or oil out, then the gas or oil is also taken from your property despite your being the rightful owner. There are many flaws in this argument even for traditional wells, but subtlety is not the forte of the New York State Senate. In the case of unconventional gas and oil, the concept completely falls apart. The well actually invades the property of a landowner forced into a drilling unit against her will. In these unconventional wells, the gas or oil would not be extracted unless the well is allowed to pass below the landowner's property. The only rationale for this law is to make extraction of hydrocarbons easier, which is, in fact, the oxymoronic mission of the NYSDEC.[8]

In the shale gas areas of Pennsylvania, the drilling operations have been under way for a number of years and the laws have been a bit more complicated. The one thing that is hard to find in Pennsylvania is a farmer who has not leased land. The reason, of course, is that until recently, most land has been leased for small sums of money and the wells that have been drilled have been small, with little disruption in terms of noise, air, or water pollution or increased traffic. Few people thought twice about leasing their land; it was seen as a way to earn a bit of spending money with little risk.

Only in the last couple of years, with the introduction of large-scale horizontal high-volume drilling, have some farmers viewed leasing as a mistake—something that could possibly drive them off the land. Although compulsory integration, similar to what is the law in New York, exists for drilling in some formations, such as the Utica Shale (specifically, "any formation below the Onondaga horizon"),[9] it does not apply to the prized Marcellus Shale because it lies above the geological marker referred to as the "Onondaga horizon."[10] Interestingly, if a farmer is integrated into a drilling unit for the Utica Shale, then she has lost her right to negotiate a lease for other formations. In the summer of 2013, Governor Corbett signed into law Act 66 of 2013,[11] which allows operators to pool leases into a single unit in all formations. This applies only to existing leases. Thus, it differs from the rules for compulsory integration of deep shale layers in Pennsylvania and the compulsory integration law in New York, which applies to all formations.

In Pennsylvania, the Clean and Green Act states that agricultural land should be assessed at the value for agricultural use rather than the fair market rate.[12] That is, the land may be more valuable if it were divided and sold as building lots in a subdivision (fair market rate) than it would be if it were used solely for agriculture. If the land is used for agricultural purposes, the Clean and Green Act requires that it be assessed on its agricultural value, which can significantly decrease a farmer's property tax bill. Placing a well on farmland removes this preferential assessment because the land is no longer being used for agriculture. In at least one case that we have investigated, compensation was written into the lease agreement to account for the fact that part of the land would now be an industrial site rather than a farm. The agreement became a problem because the entire farm lost its Clean and Green assessment, even though the compensation was only for the part of the farm that was disturbed by the drilling operation. What's more, because the well that was drilled was a test well, the farmer received no royalties that could have potentially offset the new taxes. So in the end, the farmer was forced to pay additional property taxes without full compensation.

Given complexities like these, the wide range of opinions even among farmers who have leased their land is not surprising. Some landowners are simply thrilled with the income, others like the money but have mixed feelings about the consequences of drilling, and others are very angry about the loss of their air, water, land, and way of life. In the next two chapters, we tell the stories of farmers who have suffered losses due to drilling on or near their land. These are not environmentalists; they are farmers with an ingrained skepticism of environmentalism. They don't want anyone—especially environmentalists—telling them how to farm, but they have nonetheless lost control of the use of their land because of drilling activity.

It is this intersection between drilling and farming that has the potential to affect lives outside of shale gas areas. Sometimes, when we go to the grocery store, we see produce, meat, fish, or dairy products labeled as "local," with or without the name of the individual farm on the label. But in the vast majority of cases, we really don't know where the products were produced—all we know is that they originated on a farm. If we don't know where they came from, how can we be sure our food and water are safe, given that the food could have been produced—or in the case of water, collected—in an area undergoing intensive drilling operations? On the one hand, gas drilling is similar to other heavy industry in that it has the potential to pollute air and water. However, a factory is typically not located in the middle of a cornfield or within a few feet of a pond that is the source of water for a beef cattle herd or a spring that provides drinking water for a community. But gas wells, compressor stations, processing plants, condensate tanks, and wastewater impoundments are intermingled with food production. We have seen condensate tanks venting volatile organics in a corn field, a wastewater impoundment adjacent to a field of squash, cows grazing near drilling rigs, and deer walking across drilling pads. The only honest answer to the question of whether our food and water are safe from this process is that we really don't know.

In cases of illegal dumping or leakage, the effects are catastrophic and the crops are not viable. In a large cornfield with a condensate tank at one edge, the risk may be minimal outside a small radius around the tank, but the same might not be said for a large processing facility that releases massive quantities of toxic substances into the air. Another potential for food contamination comes from practices known euphemistically as *land farming*, *land treatment*, and *land spreading*[13]—the disposal of drilling waste (drill cuttings, muds, or fluids) or wastewater on farmland that depends on soil microbes to degrade the hydrocarbons. Land farming involves multiple applications of drilling waste or wastewater to farmland, whereas land spreading and land treatment refer to a onetime application. In addition to the many types of toxic chemicals that are released from the shale during drilling and hydraulic fracturing, both drilling waste and wastewater contain radioactive compounds, mostly in the form of radium-226 and radium-228.[14] While both are hazardous substances, radium-226 is of particular concern because it can remain in the environment for thousands of years (its half-life is approximately sixteen hundred years). The states and countries allowing land farming, land treatment, and land spreading have different regulations, and the impact on agriculture has not been extensively studied. In lieu of definitive answers, some producers are rejecting milk from dairies engaged in land farming because of the high cost of testing for contaminants.[15]

With crops raised for human or animal consumption, if the effects do not kill the plants or significantly stunt their growth, then we may never know the impact on our food supply. Currently, you're unlikely to find grocery-store vegetables that have been significantly contaminated due to gas drilling, if for no other reason than the vast areas of production relative to the current footprint of gas drilling in most regions of the nation. But we have visited parts of Bradford and Washington Counties in Pennsylvania that are being intensively drilled; in some cases, the footprint of drilling approaches that of farmland. Consequently, the possible effects on farmland can only grow because the number of wells drilled as of 2013 was only a small fraction of the wells planned, even in areas that are in the middle of the shale gas boom like the one in Pennsylvania. By some estimates, up to 10 percent of US land is leased for drilling, exceeding the land mass used for growing corn and wheat.[16]

But we may never know the effects of drilling on vegetable crops, since these foods are almost never tested for chemical contaminants. In fact it is not generally in the farmer's interest to test for chemical contamination. For example, since arsenic was detected in rice products in California, some producers have been admirably open and honest about the contamination and their attempts to solve the problems. Lundberg Farms, for instance, has tested for, and published the levels of, arsenic in its rice.[17] However, the full extent of the problem is not clear. As industrial processes such as oil and gas drilling begin to take up more and more land adjacent to acres in production, more consideration must be given to the testing of these crops.

If we consider food animals, the picture changes, but not by much. Cattle can be exposed through surface spills of fracturing and drilling fluids, and wastewater, and also by contaminated water, soil, and feed. But air exposure can also be a problem, especially in farms located downwind of wastewater impoundments, condensate tanks, compressor stations, and processing plants. Air exposure may even be the leading pathway in areas such as North Dakota, where oil is being extracted unconventionally and where the gas, uncollected, is either flared or vented.[18] A particularly well-documented case of the death of two baby goats and six baby chicks on an organic goat farm illustrates the acute problems that may occur.[19] In this case, extensive air testing demonstrated elevated levels of a range of volatile organic compounds. In the case of beef herds, the animals typically go to slaughter with no chemical testing. Even testing for *E. coli* in ground meat is typically done after meat from many sources is mixed, making it impossible to track the source of contamination.[20] In dairy herds, the milk is collected and mixed with milk from many other farms—also a practice that confounds the ability to isolate the source of a potential problem.

We do know a bit more about the fate of herds with documented exposure to the products of the gas drilling industry. The most dramatic case was the death of seventeen cows in Louisiana after hydraulic fracturing fluid leaked into the pasture.[21] These previously healthy cows died within an hour, and the lesions found on necropsy suggested exposure to toxicants. Interestingly, quaternary ammonium compounds, found in the hydraulic fracturing in this case, have been described as producing similar lesions. Fortunately, these cows never made it to market; nor was their flesh rendered and sold as feed for other animals.

There are other cases, particularly wastewater impoundments that have leaked onto the pasture or into adjacent ponds used to provide drinking water for the herd. In these instances, death was not immediate, but reproductive problems were almost uniformly seen. Both beef and dairy cows typically produce one offspring per year, and the loss of production is a significant hit to a farmer's income. We have seen herds fail to produce offspring after exposure to drilling fluids and wastewater.[22] While this is not proof that the drilling fluids or the wastewater is the cause of reproductive failure, carefully controlled laboratory studies on a herd of beef cattle are not particularly easy. But farmers inadvertently set up experiments by splitting the herd into different pastures. We have several cases where part of the herd that was exposed to drilling wastewater experienced reproductive and other health problems while the unexposed part of the herd with a different source of drinking water had no changes in health. These cases provide stronger evidence that the wastewater could have caused the problem.[23]

We are, however, left with many of the same problems that we discussed in the previous section, that is, it was difficult to draw a direct link between water contamination and the health of humans and companion animals. But when dealing with farm animals, we sometimes have an exposure pathway—for example, documentation that cattle drank water contaminated by drilling wastes. The chemicals involved are far more of a problem than in contaminated well water, because the animals may be directly exposed to wastewater or hydraulic fracturing fluid whereas the contaminants in well water are diluted when such fluids leak into a freshwater aquifer. Even if all of the components of hydraulic fracturing fluid were known, the culprit or culprits may be chemicals or even bacteria extracted from the shale layers themselves or chemicals in hydraulic fracturing fluid that have undergone chemical reactions deep below the ground. Furthermore, it is notoriously difficult to trace the origin of a reproductive problem. Chemicals that work on hormonal systems can do so at very low concentrations, lower than the concentrations considered safe in drinking water (MCLs) and lower than detection levels in chemical tests.[24] Without knowing what to search for and knowing that these chemicals may be present at low levels make the problem enormously difficult and expensive to solve—certainly beyond the resources of a typical farmer. So sometimes the best we can do is study the split-herd incidents described above.

For all these reasons, we know of few cases (other than the aforementioned incident when cows were exposed to hydraulic fracturing fluid) where careful testing has been done on cattle that have been exposed to drilling contaminants. But consider the motivation for testing. No farmer wants her farm to be thought of as the one that is raising cattle using contaminated water—an understandable attitude. Perhaps it is better just to move on and hope the problem goes away next year. This approach may sound somewhat lackadaisical, and it does not help those of us studying these problems, but it may actually be a reasonable strategy for the farmer. For the most part, chemical toxicants have a measurable lifetime in the cow's body, and if you wait long enough, they will all be excreted, with the possible exception of the metals strontium[25] and radium-226,[26] both having a long half-life in bone tissue. So if the cows are not sent to the slaughterhouse or the renderer and do reproduce the next year, perhaps all is well. With any luck, the problem will go away and subsequent generations will not be exposed to any toxic chemicals.

Maybe, maybe not. Not only do we have very little knowledge about what toxicants may be in these cows' bodies, but even if we did know, we still know little about how long an individual chemical remains in the body. Nor do we know if any of these compounds have epigenetic effects (heritable changes in DNA, for example, methylation). Most research to date has focused on antibiotics and pesticides. Knowing how long an antibiotic stays in the body can provide an indication of a safe interval to allow between administering the antibiotic and sending the cow to slaughter. With drilling chemicals, the best that can be done is to make educated guesses. We are currently aware of only one instance when beef cattle were quarantined following exposure to drilling wastewater.[27] The length of the quarantine was not predicated on hard science, but was a guess based on the herd's exposure to only some of the chemicals in the wastewater (volatile and semivolatile organic compounds were not included in the analysis of the wastewater) and how similar compounds are excreted. Nevertheless, the quarantine might actually be considered a success of the regulatory system because something was done. In other cases, cattle have moved on to slaughter and rendering without further testing.

As things stand, there are no incentives to report or study food safety issues associated with gas drilling. A farmer who has leased his land wants to continue farming and reap the profits from the gas well. If a spill occurs or if water is contaminated, the farmer can suffer, but he may suffer even more if word gets out that his animals may have been exposed to toxic chemicals.

Although the issue is now a gray area, the ramifications can be even greater for an organic farmer, who may lose organic certification because of possible contamination. Organic standards are set by the National Organic Program of the US Department of Agriculture and include setbacks and buffers from industrial activity.[28] Individual certifiers control the actual enforcement, and what constitutes an adequate buffer zone is determined on a case-by-case basis, adding a layer of ambiguity to the organic certification.

So in both organic farms and the more conventional farms, the financial incentives are all stacked toward keeping quiet about any possible contamination. Putting it in this context is a bit sterile, since we can only assume that most farmers want to produce products that are fresh and healthy. The problem, however, is more complicated and confusing. The farmers to whom we have spoken and who have had instances of water contamination on their farm have been told by either the drilling companies or state regulators that there was no problem: the wastewater leaked into the pond from which the cows drink, but nothing in the wastewater can cause a problem. While the authority figure pronouncing the water safe may in fact be correct, without complete testing it is impossible to know for sure. Under these circumstances, it is easy to send animals on to slaughter without a second thought.

We do not know the extent of the problem of land, water, and air contamination from unconventional drilling operations, but it can only grow as drilling expands. What we do know is that drilling fluids, fracturing fluids, wastewater, and air contaminants released during drilling

operations contain chemicals that are human carcinogens or are suspected human carcinogens and that consequently, crops from exposed
fields; milk, meat, and eggs from exposed animals; and fish from exposed
waterways should not be made available for human consumption.

The cows that were exposed to hydraulic fracturing fluid in Louisiana
and died within an hour were buried shortly afterward. This is not the
usual fate of cows that die or are too sick to be sent to slaughter; these
animals are usually sent to a renderer. Animals exposed to drilling fluids,
wastewater, or contaminated drinking water can be sent to rendering
plants without further testing. But as discussed, for crops grown on
farms shared with drilling operations and cattle exposed to drilling
contaminants and sent to slaughter, we don't know the extent of the
problem. Simply stating over and over that no problem exists does not
make it so.

Perhaps if cows could swim, the FDA would be monitoring our milk
and meat to be sure these foods were safe for human consumption. Currently, the FDA monitors seafood after major oil spills by using specific
protocols to determine food safety.[29] As with onshore unconventional
fossil fuel extraction, we don't know the identities of all the chemicals
used for offshore drilling (and may never know). Yet, one of the groups
of compounds that the FDA, EPA, and NOAA (National Oceanic and
Atmospheric Administration) have chosen for analysis is the PAHs
(polycyclic aromatic hydrocarbons), perhaps the most studied and most
persistent compounds found in petroleum mixtures.[30] PAHs are a human health concern because of their potential carcinogenic, mutagenic,
and teratogenic effects[31] and because exposure during pregnancy is associated with adverse effects on birth and early childhood development.[32] As PAHs are components of drilling and fracturing fluid[33] and
are also found in wastewater,[34] they could be similarly used to monitor
our crops, meat, eggs, and dairy products following contamination
events on land.

In addition to PAHs, it would be prudent to monitor our food supply for radium-226, which is found in both drilling waste and wastewater. The presence of radium-226 in these wastes is of great concern for
a number of reasons. Besides having a very long half-life, radium-226

can be absorbed by both plants and animals and bioaccumulates in some fish and aquatic plants; people who eat contaminated food products may then be exposed to radium-226.[35] In particular, this element replaces calcium in the bones of animals, including humans, and can cause cancer.[36] The vast volumes of wastewater are disposed of in a number of ways (see the appendix, "A Primer on Gas Drilling"), including treatment at wastewater-treatment facilities, which discharge into streams and public drinking-water supplies. A recent study reported levels of radium-226 in stream sediments near an oil and gas wastewater-treatment facility that were approximately two hundred times higher than background levels[37] and more than two times above US regulatory levels.[38]

Currently, little information is available on what this means for the drinking water and food of people and animals living near such facilities, and for people and animals living in areas where *untreated* wastewater has been spilled on farmlands, dumped into streams, and spread on roads. But we believe that no harm can come of tracking and monitoring our food and water sourced from intensively drilled areas for PAHs and radium-226. If, indeed, all is well, then the public will be reassured. If, however, exposure pathways and specific chemicals are identified, then it may be possible to find ways to mitigate the problem.

Meanwhile, we shouldn't wait until all the science is in before we decide to protect the public's health. In the early 1990s, nuanced approaches to risk management were successful in preventing an outbreak of bovine spongiform encephalopathy ("mad cow disease") and variant Creutzfeldt-Jakob disease in the United States.[39] These actions prove that we *can* make a careful analysis of risk with incomplete data sets and prevent such public health disasters as we have seen with tobacco use and may yet see in areas undergoing unconventional fossil fuel extraction.

Beyond worries of food safety, the larger issue looming before farmers in several drought-stricken, intensively drilled states in the West and Southwest is whether they will be able to farm in the future.[40] In these states, farmers are competing with the fossil fuel industry for a rapidly dwindling water supply: in Colorado, more than 90 percent of unconventional wells were hydraulically fractured in extremely high water stress areas while in Texas, more than 50 percent of wells were hydraulically fractured in high or extremely high water stress areas.[41] Without water, farmers are forced to fallow fields that would otherwise be productive, or lease the land to the oil and gas companies. Either way, less food is produced. If the fossil fuel industry continues to use the water that our nation's farmers so desperately depend on, we will be asking ourselves not how safe is our food, but where will our food come from?

In chapters 6 and 7, we illustrate the problems associated with farming in intensively drilled areas with the stories of two farm families raising cattle in Pennsylvania. These are people who have lived in the same area since they were born and who have long histories of farming. When they tell us that their herd's health has changed since drilling began, they mean that the health of their cattle has been the same for many years but has dramatically changed within a few short years. These farmers are not environmental activists—they are simply good people yearning for respect and acknowledgment of the problems that they have endured during the last few years.

SIX

MARY AND CHARLIE
Quarantined Cattle

The Jamesons' farm sits six miles east of the Grand Canyon of Pennsylvania,[1] where Mary Jameson's father kept concession stands for thirty years. Mary doesn't come from farming stock, except for an uncle who was a farmer—"and that doesn't count for much," according to his niece. It's Mary's husband, Charlie, who has farming in his blood: he took his first breath up the road on his father's farm, where the business was dairy cattle and potatoes. His mother sold her farm to Charlie for one dollar at a time when the farm was 73 acres with fourteen little red outbuildings; the farm now consists of 530 acres, with the Jamesons' son Joe on the upper farm and Charlie and Mary on the lower farm.

Charlie's original intention was to run a gentleman's farm, but soon after he acquired thirty high-grade cows, the number in his herd ballooned to ninety. Charlie, as full-time dairyman, and Mary, as part-time help on weekends, kept the dairy business going for over thirty years. After they stopped sending milk, they continued to sell hay and put up corn, but soon threw in a few head of beef cattle, just to keep Charlie busy. Those few head gradually grew to over thirty, the number the Jamesons grazed before the gas drilling rig made its presence known in their backyard.

And it is literally in their backyard. Their driveway is now the access road, with trucks rumbling in and out just feet from their kitchen window. Facing me at the kitchen table, Charlie interrupted my questions to ask if I have seen the bank leading up to the well pad; he wanted me to see how close it is to the house and how it slopes right down to his barn.

I visited the Jamesons in October 2011, almost a year and a half after a wastewater spill into their grazing pasture led to the PADEP-ordered quarantine of most of their beef cattle and the subsequent loss of calves in the following breeding season. Of all the things that have happened on this farm, the placement of the well pad so close to his house, barn, and cattle pasture seemed to rankle Charlie the most. To me—an outsider and a nonfarmer—this looked small compared to the major cost of the herd quarantine and the loss of calves and many acres of pastureland and hay fields.

"That's all we got to look at is that doggone bank and the well pad they put there," Charlie said. "They give you a song and dance that they will only be there a couple years and then it will all be put back to its natural state. Well! That's gonna stay like that indefinitely. It came right up next to our shed here, and I just took my little farm loader and opened it up a little bit so I could get around that."

I stared at the banks, and the banks stared back, unmowed and untrimmed. "So they're supposed to take care of all that?" I asked.

Both farmers snickered. "Especially if they're in your backyard!" Charlie answered. "If it's out in the back forty, where nobody sees it, I can understand—maybe not mow it. But right here, they should keep it tidy a little bit, especially [with] people with hay fever."

Charlie dropped his gaze to the table and said, "We can't get 'em to do anything."

To demonstrate what their farm looked like before drilling, Mary showed me a large framed aerial color photo of the farmhouse, barns, shed, cattle pasture, and cattle. Behind the barns and shed was pastureland, gently sloping upward and divided by a stand of trees with a dirt road running alongside. I noticed the missing stand of trees and what was once the gentle hill behind the barn, now built up by thirty feet. The pasture had been ripped apart for transmission pipelines that will trespass across the property and up to an adjoining well at a higher elevation, above the airport. That means more fencing to be interrupted and rebuilt. Because of the constant upheaval on their farm, they keep a six-strand barbed-wire fence on hand.

The farmers lost a pasture, a gravity-fed manure system, and a beautiful view from their house and from the top of the hill. The cattle lost continuous grazing land.

But it's how they've been mistreated that gets under the skin of both farmers—ignored by drillers who call themselves neighbors. A request for compensation for a cattle chute to manage the bull calves held under quarantine was refused, and a demand to have the herd replaced was ignored. Recently, the company voluntarily raised the issue of compensation for the beef herd. Mary's response: "A dollar late and a day short! I have turned that over to our attorney. That 'til it's all said and done will take years—maybe more than we have. The last person they paid off had to sign a gag restriction. They won't get that from us. Any story that I have given [to the media] has not been nasty but rather reaching for answers and attempting to educate people as to what they need to look out for."

These were not the happy farmers to which the gas industry proudly refers—the ones with the new barn, content cows, new fences, and new stake on life. I wondered if Charlie and Mary were ever happy with the drillers. Did the Jamesons know what they were getting into when they leased? Mary answered, "No, no, no. We were just gonna help pay the taxes." And if they could do it over again, would they? They both responded at the same time: Mary didn't think so. She's had enough to take care of, she said, she didn't need this. Charlie was more direct, more emphatic. He stiffened and looked me straight in the eye: "No. Absolutely, no." Years ago, they explained, leasing helped pay the taxes, but there was deep regret in their voices and a desire to explain more. Charlie described how a landsman first came around in 2000 and asked if they wanted to lease their land for $1 per acre.

"Well, that sounded pretty good then. So we said, 'OK, why not?' You know, well, I mean, you got nothing to lose, right?" To emphasize the absurdity of this situation, Charlie pointed to the well pad, grinned, and asked again, "Right?" After ten years,[2] the landsman returned and offered to double the leasing rate to $2 per acre, which the Jamesons accepted. Shaking his pencil at the well pad area, Charlie said, "And that's what they put that on: a two-dollar-an-acre lease." He let the pencil fall to the table. "We hung ourselves."

According to the farmers, almost everybody in the county was leased at that point, "one way or another." The few who didn't gobble up the $1- and $2-per-acre leases held out for the $5,000-per-acre leases.

Charlie added, "So they're the only ones who are winning, I guess, if there's a win to it."

I asked about the well location site fee; did that help? Charlie grimaced before answering, "They take a lot of ground. And they only pay fifteen thousand dollars to be tied up, how long? Maybe fifteen, maybe a hundred years. You know, that's not compensation enough." Did their lease give them any say on where the well would be located? According to the lease, this is supposed to be negotiable. But when the Jamesons pressed the issue, they began to fear they would not receive their $15,000 site fee, so they backed down. But a neighbor didn't, and so far she has not received her site fee. Mary explained that there is no specific clause in their lease stating that the site fee must be paid. In fact, leases sometimes include a site fee clause, but it's often conditional and goes unpaid.

Were these farmers ever told what might happen? No, they said, they were not. "We never realized that all this could explode like this," Charlie said, shaking his head. They noted that in their neighborhood, a lot of real estate is for sale—mostly houses—not selling because of problems obtaining mortgages.

According to the Jamesons, the landsmen were out to get everyone "leased up" and became angry and began yelling if the farmers questioned anything. But a year ago, a landsman offered them $800 an acre to put a seven- or eight-acre freshwater impoundment on a part of their land located across the road from the cow pastures and barn. Mary and Charlie refused out of concern for their neighbors as well as the loss of more of their land, but this particular landsman wasn't upset by their reply. Charlie, who had his chair rocked back from the table while Mary was talking, drew back in and assumed an elfish grin. "Well," he said, "that was one of the most sincere people they sent around; that landsman said he wouldn't allow it to be put on his ground!"

On July 1, 2010, the PADEP issued a press release: wastewater from a drilling site had leaked into an adjacent cow pasture on a beef cattle farm.[3] Minerals and metals were found, including strontium, and the entire herd, save two bulls, was placed on quarantine.

Several things bothered me about this press release. First, there was nearly a two-month gap between the time the Jamesons' quarantine was instituted on May 5, 2010, and the time it was reported to the public. Second, there was no mention of tests for radioactivity or organic compounds. This was a food safety issue, and I had some basic questions. Did the drilling company provide the PADEP with a list of the drilling muds and hydraulic fracturing fluids that were used? Was the wastewater tested for these chemicals as well as others released from the shale during fracturing, such as radioactive compounds and the carcinogen benzene? Were the quarantine recommendations based on solid knowledge of the chemicals that are often found in shale gas wastewater?

I immediately called the PADEP and was connected to the animal health division. After several calls and emails, I learned that the Jamesons' quarantine had developed into a legal matter, and details of this case could not be discussed with anyone. Apparently, the case arose from the drilling company's questioning of the legality of the quarantine. This seemed strange to me, since it was the farmers, not the drilling company, who stood to lose the most financially. Yet no one, including the drilling company, was offering any compensation to Mary and Charlie. By year's end, the case was resolved, and the quarantine remained in place.

Because of my veterinary and pharmacology background, I contacted the Food Animal Residue Avoidance Databank (FARAD),[4] the group advising PADEP on the Jamesons' quarantine guidelines. Unfortunately, the initial response was that unless I was the attending veterinarian, my questions would not be answered. Surely, I thought, FARAD would answer general questions from a concerned veterinarian. So I sent an email listing several chemicals commonly occurring in drilling wastewater—chemicals such as radon, radium-226, arsenic, barium, cadmium, lead, mercury, strontium, benzene, toluene, xylene, diesel fuel, kerosene, naphthalene, methylene, ethylene glycol, and hydrochloric acid, and I asked several questions:

- How are recommendations made in cases where the amount of chemical consumed is unclear?
- How are recommendations made in cases where half-life values (the time it takes for half of the chemical to be eliminated from

the body) and withdrawal times (the time an animal is held from slaughter after the last exposure to a chemical or medication) have not been previously determined for the affected species?

• Through negligence, accidents, and lack of regulations, these chemicals, many of which are highly toxic and should have no "safe" level in food, will enter our food supply and cause severe, insidious long-term human and animal health problems. How can this problem be addressed?

The response from FARAD was simple: "We do not answer 'general questions.'" The agency referred me to a state veterinarian working in conjunction with a state diagnostic laboratory, or someone at a veterinary school. After several additional emails, I heard from one of FARAD's codirectors, who advised on quarantine guidelines. He was lamenting his inability to answer my questions due to a lack of federal funding, specifically that related to chemical contamination.

I first spoke with Mary in January 2011, when the Jameson herd was eight months into the quarantine. Mary mentioned that due to the quarantine, she and Charlie would be forced to keep the bull calves for two years and that the bulls were hard to handle even with a cattle chute. Mary estimated that they had lost more than $10,000 but were not pursuing a lawsuit as they hoped they would make this money back in royalty payments once the wells were actively producing. Nevertheless, six head had gone to slaughter—as either adults after six months' quarantine or yearlings after eight months' quarantine. The cows that did not become pregnant were sent to auction. Only one cow of these had anything wrong with it—a cancer in the eye. Mary was concerned about this cow, so she specifically asked that the carcass be checked at the slaughterhouse to see if the cancer spread (it had not). Afraid that no one would purchase her cows because everyone knew what had happened on their farm, Mary wasn't looking forward to the auction. Despite her fears, the cattle were purchased and sent on to slaughter, and she was happy with what she was paid for each carcass.

Was the wastewater impoundment still on the Jamesons' property?

Soon after the quarantine was instituted, the drillers removed the impoundment and now store wastewater in very large trailer trucks on Mary and Charlie's property and at another site where a wastewater impoundment leaked.

Exposure of wildlife, especially deer, to wastewater seemed to bother Mary much more than her cows being exposed and going on to slaughter. Deer were always on the well pad, especially when the impoundment was there, and it was impossible to keep them off. In a later interview, Mary mentioned two men who regularly hunted on their farmland and continued to do so after the Jamesons' well was drilled and hydraulically fractured. The men shot a small and a large deer and became ill with vomiting and diarrhea after cooking the meat for themselves, and later for friends—where everyone became severely ill. They also noted that their cats and dogs wouldn't touch the meat, cooked or raw.

Mary had ten packages of the meat in her freezer, including the liver from one of the deer, and was hoping that I could have it tested. She had tried to have it tested but was told that legally she couldn't test the meat because it belonged to the Pennsylvania Game Commission, and the commission couldn't test the meat because there was no chain of custody, that is, no written documentation of the source of the meat.

Mary's quandary of who should test her deer meat raised many questions regarding testing of cattle in situations where known exposures have occurred. Cows that were exposed to toxic chemicals from shale gas wastewater, that were not tested before or after slaughter, and that were held from slaughter based on incomplete testing (estimated withdrawal times for only one contaminant) would produce flesh that would be packaged and eaten alongside the flesh of other cows that had no such exposure, and whose rendered flesh would be fed to chickens and pigs, made into pet food, and gain entrance into our food supply, as well as that of our pets.

These concerns are also on the mind of the public and are the topic of intense debate. How safe are the meat, eggs, dairy products, and vegetable crops from farms where known exposures have occurred and from farms downstream and downwind of the exposure?

The answer is that without complete testing, without many more dollars targeted to food safety research specifically related to chemical contamination from shale gas operations, we will never know. And as long as we don't know, the public health may be at risk.

Midway through our interview in October 2011, Mary disappeared and returned with a stack of photos. She spread them on the table, and Charlie picked out several and passed them to me. They were photos of the well pad during hydraulic fracturing.

In the photos, everything was jumbled and squeezed together, even to the edges of the pad. From a distance the pad looked like a dump, like vehicles of all sorts randomly thrown together. It reminded me of a child's room: a pile of red, yellow, blue, and white blocks left behind after playtime, or the Rush Hour game, where all the cars and trucks sit on the board with no place to move. On closer inspection, I saw that many kinds of vehicles were represented, including a bulldozer, chemical tanks lined up in tight rows, white pickup trucks and vans, a hot-lunch truck, and the iconic water and sand trucks that all too often pass me on the highways. At the center was the wellhead, looking like a giant octopus, its arms the lines that are used to pump the pressurized water and chemicals deep down into the earth. Charlie described the vehicles and equipment on the pad as being so tightly packed that no one could walk up there. Their two-acre well pad (later expanded to three acres) had become the parking lot from hell.

While I studied the photos, I realized that this interview was making the Jamesons relive everything, and for that I was sorry. But they wanted me to know exactly what they endured, and to experience what it felt like to have their property invaded. Most of all, they wanted others to benefit from the mistakes they had made.

This first shale gas well sits directly behind their barn and next to their cow pasture. It was drilled in October 2009, was hydraulically fractured from January to April 2010, and reaches at least six thousand feet straight down into the earth. From there, it turns and runs horizontally to the northwest as far as it can, which is approximately another six thousand feet, butting up against unleased state forest land. Five more wells are planned, but the Jamesons were not told exactly when the others would be drilled.

I brought a paper map showing the permitted gas wells within ten miles of their home, according to the most current PADEP well data. On the map, Mary and Charlie's farm was a blue teardrop completely surrounded by red balloons with black dots, representing gas wells on each pad. On the electronic version of the map, I zoomed in many times before the blue teardrop stood alone untouched by the red bubbles, and this was the first version I showed them, the one where all of the more than four hundred wells are still on the page. Zooming in further, the bubbles began to separate, and outlines of bubbles began to emerge behind what initially appeared as just one bubble, as if they were many soldiers standing toe to heel.

We were down to twenty-five bubbles, with each bubble representing one to six gas wells. I asked about several nearby bubbles that also bear their name. One of these is on a cousin's land, they explained, located a little over a mile south of them, but Mary and Charlie were unsure of exactly how many wells sat on this pad. After further zooming in, we discovered that there are two Marcellus wells here: a vertical—drilled approximately six months after theirs—and a horizontal that has yet to be drilled. I asked about the other well bearing their name and located approximately one-half mile to the east of them. This well will be placed on their upper farm, they said, despite their objections and despite this being their best farmland. "We're trying to get 'em to relocate that well," Charlie said. "We're looking for some top brass to talk to, to get 'em to do it, because we've had enough of it. You'd think with all that has happened to this well [the one within view of their kitchen window], they'd say, 'Mr. Jameson, you've had a lot of complications. We'll put it on your neighbor's ground. Thank you!'" Charlie laughed at the thought of this, as if this could, or would ever happen.

Air. Water. Soil. These are the three things I think about when associating exposures with how people and their animals become ill. In the Jamesons' case, the exposure seemed pretty clear-cut: wastewater leaked into the cow pasture, hoofprints were found in the flooded area, and as cows are attracted to salt, and the wastewater was heavily laden with salts, state health officials assumed the cows drank the toxic water.[5] But there was more: there were interactions that I hadn't considered initially, and they would become important once I received all the known test results.

After talking inside, Charlie invited me to tour the pad, to see the pasture and the cattle, to get a lay of the land. As we walked up the hill to the pad, we stepped over a metal grate between the shed and the Jamesons' big red barn, placed by the drilling company to direct runoff from the pad. We then climbed steeply and continued up the bank to the pad area. In stark contrast to the photos taken during hydraulic fracturing, the pad was deserted except for two red pickup trucks parked side by side, and two men. The men waved to Charlie and headed out toward where pipeline was being laid; Charlie said that they were inspecting the line. According to Mary, Charlie was always up on the pad, watching the workers, talking with them, asking questions. Nothing slipped by him. I watched Charlie, still cheerful and friendly to these workers in the face of all that has happened on his farm and all the losses he has taken as a result of their disruption of his land, and I understood why they respected him.

The wellhead, condensate tank, and compressor stood silent, like soldiers guarding the pad. Because the well was not actively producing, the pad was deathly quiet. At the far edge of the pad, Charlie pointed to where the drilling muds pit had been located, the liner now ripped out and removed, the top layer of soil extracted. We stood at the edge of the pad facing the cow pasture, the lower barns and a long view of this peaceful, picturesque valley. The cattle, their numbers dropped by seven since drilling began, grazed at the far end of this twenty-acre pasture that will be divided and gated after the pipeline is placed. I asked about the cattle's water sources, and the Jamesons pointed to the creek that originates from springs lying above and below the well pad, and to a pond below the well pad, which also spills into the creek. Between where we stood and where the cattle grazed, the bank of the pad drops down to a level one-acre rectangle of uncut grass before the land crosses under a fence and gently slopes down into the pasture and to the creek and the pond.

This rectangle began its life on the Jameson farm as a freshwater impoundment, a place to store millions of gallons of water used during high-volume hydraulic fracturing, but was quickly transformed into a holding pond for wastewater—whatever flows back to the surface during and after hydraulic fracturing operations have occurred. Amounts returning to the surface may be less than 30 percent to more than 70 percent of the original fluids injected into the shale,[6] and are contaminated by chemical additives as well as naturally occurring substances normally found in the shale such as heavy metals, volatile organics, and radioactive compounds.

A few months before they reported the wastewater leak to the PADEP and the drilling company, Mary and Charlie had noticed several dark spots on the bank of the impoundment alongside the pasture. At first they thought it was groundwater seeping into the pasture, but over the coming weeks, they noticed the spots expanding and the adjacent grass dying. By the time they ventured onto the pasture, hydraulic fracturing had ended and there was no one on the pad. It was May Day 2010, and the farmers found themselves ankle-deep in wastewater and surrounded by burnt grass. Hoofprints covered the flooded area, estimated by Charlie and Mary to be more than one-half acre. The water was as deep as twenty inches in some spots and would eventually take the drillers three days to pump and remove. The Jamesons later learned that the liners of both the wastewater impoundment and the drilling muds pit had torn, and that the rupture in the impoundment liner had caused the contaminated waste to burst through the wall and into the pasture where their cows grazed. Except for their two bulls, the Jamesons' entire herd was exposed to the wastewater leakage for as long as it had been occurring, likely two months or more.

On the PADEP website, I skimmed the Notice Of Violation dataset until I found the Jamesons' records and, in the process, discovered that ruptured, torn, and leaky liners are not unusual. Under each of the four violations issued, there were comments, which shed more light on what had happened. According to the record, because it was the Jamesons' daughter who first contacted the PADEP, the drilling company was charged with failure to notify the agency. The company also failed to line the impoundment properly: subsequent pressure testing of the liner revealed a failed patch, which meant a loss of the liner's integrity. Because the spring and farm pond were located downgradient from the leaky impoundment, creating the potential to pollute these surface waters, this was a violation of Pennsylvania's Clean Streams Law. Finally, because the drilling company had mismanaged its residual waste, allowing the wastewater to contaminate the cow pasture, the company was charged with violating the Pennsylvania Oil and Gas Act 223.[7]

To Charlie and Mary's credit, they didn't wait for the water flooding their cow pasture to be tested and confirmed as contaminated with "dangerous chemicals and metals" (according to the PADEP press release)[8] before they quarantined their herd. Of all the known contaminants to which the Jamesons' cattle were exposed, strontium was of most concern to the PADEP and was the reason the quarantine was placed. Strontium can be toxic to both animals and people because it replaces the calcium in bones, especially those of the young, and it may take years to be eliminated from bone tissue.[9] The quarantine hold times (the length of time the cattle are held before going to slaughter) were based on estimates of how long strontium would remain in a cow's body. Of greater concern, however, are the *unknown* chemicals to which these cattle may have been exposed, including toxic substances used as fracturing fluid additives, such as 2-butoxyethanol, glutaraldehyde, and tetramethylammonium chloride. Neither the public, who would consume the meat from these cows, nor the Jamesons, who would subsequently pay for necropsies to determine what was killing their cattle, were told what chemicals were used during drilling and hydraulic fracturing. For unknown reasons, testing for organic compounds was not done on the wastewater to which these cows were exposed.

When I asked the Jamesons if their tap water has been affected, they told me that initially it ran cloudy, then would clear immediately. But lately it has been staying cloudy longer. Despite that, Charlie and Mary were more concerned with the cattle's water than with their own. Tests done on their well water before and after drilling yielded no significant findings, although no testing was done for organic compounds. However, the cattle's sources of water—the spring, the creek, and the pond— were not tested before drilling began, and if it were not for the leaky impoundment, testing may never have been done on the cattle's water. Like the Jamesons' well water, no abnormal results appeared.

In addition to water tests, the PADEP also ordered the soil to be tested, but again failed to check for organic compounds. When compared to background samples, soil tests done on the contaminated cow pasture revealed high levels of chloride, sulfate, sodium and strontium. In an attempt to return the cow pasture to what it once was, approximately twelve inches of topsoil were removed, according to Mary and Charlie. On retesting, the sulfate concentrations in the confirmation sample remained stubbornly high—nearly the same as before the attempt at remediation—literally three times higher than the sulfate normally found in the soil.

Veterinary and music students know that all cows eat grass. But cows also eat soil. As Mary and Charlie's cows were exposed to high sulfate in the soil for over a year, the high sulfate in the soil could also mean that the herd was exposed to high sulfate in the grass. I wondered if the sulfate could be acting directly or indirectly to cause some of the reproductive problems that the Jamesons were having with their cattle. For answers, I turned to local animal and soil scientists and learned that in general, higher levels of sulfate in the soil would mean higher levels of sulfate in the grass, and that because sulfur is chemically similar to selenium, too much of one could mean a decrease in the absorption of the other.[10]

Why be concerned with selenium? Selenium needs to be at just the right level in the body, or things go wrong reproductively: both too much and too little will cause cows to abort and calves to be born dead or weak.[11] For more than thirty years tending dairy cattle and for more than twenty years raising beef, the Jamesons had never thought about selenium levels: whatever their herd was getting in the grass must be perfect because their cows had always been healthy, with little or no loss of calves.

Things started going very wrong for their cattle soon after Charlie and Mary discovered wastewater in their cow pasture on May Day 2010. On that very day, a three-year-old cow aborted, and a few days later, several cows blocked their calves from nursing, leading to the death of one of the calves.[12] For the Jamesons, such death and behavior in their herd were unusual, and they made a mental note of it. But these losses were nothing compared to what they would endure the following season, the second living with a shale gas well behind the barn.

As we walked off the well pad on our October 2011 visit, Charlie pointed to his herd, also on the move, the calves trailing the adults single file behind the boss cow. I was far away but close enough to discern that the last six animals are smaller, and that these must be the survivors, the only calves remaining from last season, where eleven out of a total of seventeen calves were lost. I wondered what happened to the others. Three of these calves died between one and two months of age, withering away, unable to stand or to take nourishment. Mary and Charlie described pulling dead calves—seven—and said that one calf was born alive but was too ill to suckle. All of the dams (mothers) of these calves were directly exposed to the chemicals in the wastewater, and the contaminated soil and grass, and their calves indirectly so, in utero. The wastewater chemicals potentially included drilling and hydraulic fracturing fluid additives as well as the organic compounds, heavy metals, and radioactive elements brought to the surface during hydraulic fracturing. Searching for answers, the Jamesons followed the advice of the state veterinarian and sent the ill calf and a stillborn calf for necropsy.

The necropsy report on the Jamesons' calves was most remarkable for what it didn't include rather than what it did. Surprisingly, there was no mention of this herd's recent exposure to shale gas wastewater and to the subsequent quarantine—it was as if it didn't happen. Because the wastewater was analyzed for inorganics, this presented an unusual opportunity to screen the livers of both calves for all of the specific minerals and metals that had seeped into the cattle's pasture. While some chemicals were tested, others—including barium, potassium, sodium, fluoride, chloride, sulfate, and strontium—were not. It is especially hard to understand why strontium was not tested: strontium was the reason this herd had been quarantined, the reason Mary and Charlie had lost thousands of dollars, and the reason people were asking questions about the safety of their meat. By being chemically similar to calcium, strontium can replace calcium in the body and, in so doing, poses a serious threat to young growing animals, including the human variety.[13]

Vitamin E and selenium levels were checked, and both calves had low levels. Whatever the cause, low levels of vitamin E and selenium are fairly common in beef cattle in Pennsylvania and are a likely reason for the high rate of stillborn calves in this herd. Case closed, end of discussion? I didn't think so. The necropsy report failed to answer the big question that arose from these results, the question that desperately needed to be answered: what caused the low levels of vitamin E and selenium on a farm that has had very low calf losses for over fifty years and has never supplemented the herd? Typically, something has to change to tip healthy cattle over the edge—perhaps the management, or maybe a bad winter, or bad forage.

But according to Mary and Charlie, none of these things had changed. The only things that did change were the presence of a shale gas well—less than a hundred feet from their barn door—and a wastewater impoundment, adjacent to their pasture and within two hundred feet from the creek and pond where their cattle drink. As mentioned, the connection to the wastewater exposure and the low selenium levels was most likely the interaction between selenium and sulfate. The word *interaction* is key because we must be concerned not only with the interactions between the individual chemicals associated with the drilling process, but also with the interactions between these chemicals in the body and, as in Mary and Charlie's herd, the interactions between these chemicals and other substances found in the environment.

Back in Mary and Charlie's kitchen, we talked again about the eleven calves they had lost. The death that frustrated these farmers the most was that of the calf that was too weak to suckle and never received any colostrum (first milk produced by the dam that contains antibodies and nutrients), the calf they brought in from the pasture and tried to save but couldn't, the calf that was euthanized at less than a week old for necropsy and diagnosed with *E. coli* septicemia. We talked about how calves become infected with *E. coli*. I asked if the dam was ill, if the placenta or the umbilical cord was infected, if the calf had any wounds, how clean the barn was. They had thought of all these things and reviewed them endless times. Everything was fine, they said, except this calf had absolutely no suckle reflex.

Septicemia is defined as the presence of disease-producing organisms or their toxins in the blood, and *E. coli* is the most common bacterial cause of septicemia in calves. Mary and Charlie understand that because their calf had a poor suckle reflex, it likely didn't receive enough colostrum from the dam and was more susceptible to infections. But because the calf's immunoglobulin G levels were not checked, they'll never know for sure. What they do know is that septicemia and a high incidence of calf deaths on a well-kept farm with good husbandry are highly unusual; what they don't know is exactly which chemicals were used to drill and hydraulically fracture the shale gas well on their farm, and if any of these chemicals acted as immunosuppressants to cause the problems they experienced. Can immunity be affected by gas drilling operations? While there are no definitive answers, one study estimates that nearly 40 percent of the known chemicals used in drilling and hydraulic fracturing for gas may cause immunosuppression.[14]

There was another interesting finding on the necropsy report. The stillborn calf also suffered from goiter, an enlargement of the thyroid gland. This is not a common diagnosis in cows or calves, so why might it appear in this case? More than a third of the known chemicals used in drilling and hydraulic fracturing for gas may cause endocrine disruption,[15] and this diagnosis may be a manifestation of such an exposure in this herd.

I asked the Jamesons if they had approached the drilling company to inquire about the exact chemicals used during drilling and hydraulic fracturing. Charlie said they hadn't, but he had heard that anyone can, and the drilling company would provide the names of the chemicals. Later I checked the industry website, fracfocus.org, billed as the site where one can get information about the chemicals used at each well (that is, only nonproprietary chemicals, and only after the hydraulic fracturing is complete and too late to use for predrilling testing). No information was provided for the Jameson well.

We talked about neighbors, about farming, about the land. After their experiences with just one shale gas well, these farmers were rightly worried about the consequences of five more. After watching the US Department of Energy hearing held in Washington County in 2011, Charlie and Mary said they were amazed how people stepped forward to tell their woes, how one woman said she couldn't sit on her front porch anymore because she's right next to a compressor station.

"Yes, this is terrible," Charlie said. "After they get all this going [the full build-out of wells], are we gonna lose our vegetation? That's my question. What do you think? Do you think we're gonna lose our leaves, everything? Is this gonna be barren ground? Is this gonna be like the coal regions of Pennsylvania?"

He looked straight at me, and it was clear he wanted an answer immediately. It was something he had been thinking about for a while, something he found deeply disturbing. But he threw me off balance—I wasn't prepared for this. I'm more comfortable talking about animal sickness and death.

"I don't know" is all I could muster.

Charlie hadn't finished his question. "Eventually this is gonna hit our atmosphere. It won't happen overnight. But eventually, it [the vegetation, the soil] will all be dead. It's a possibility, right?"

I mentioned a study in West Virginia, where application of hydraulic fracturing fluids to a forest severely affected the trees and ground vegetation.[16] I described several cases in Colorado, North Dakota, and Pennsylvania where vegetation was killed in areas where gas came up to the surface along fault lines and fracture lines after hydraulic fracturing, and along ruptured pipelines.

Charlie shook his head and said that he had heard of people being told to move away when their water became contaminated. I've heard this many times, too, and I told Mary and Charlie that I *know* people who have moved several times and people who are planning to move. I told the Jamesons that sometimes people stay, despite their doctors' telling them to move. They stay because they can't bear to leave their homes, and sometimes they will stay in their homes with the windows shut and will not go out.

There was a long silence between us—we had covered a lot of ground, and it seemed that we had all learned something from each other today. Now, I had no more questions, and the Jamesons needed to attend to their herd. As I was preparing to leave, Charlie mentioned that I should see the Grand Canyon of Pennsylvania while I was in the area. I was anxious to move on to my next interview, but his enthusiasm was contagious. He described how people come from all over to see the canyon and there was no way that I could visit the area and not see it. How could I resist? It was probably just what I needed to cheer me up after hearing their story, so I headed off to see this natural wonder.

On the way, I observed gas pipelines being laid every few hundred feet, randomly crisscrossing the road. It seemed that no part of Tioga County would be untouched. I later would have a look at the permits issued in the area and the plans for drilling, and indeed, no area is to be untouched. However, on reaching Pine Creek Gorge, the beautiful area known as the Grand Canyon of Pennsylvania, I was transported to another place and time. Like the gorges in my beloved Finger Lakes region of New York, this spectacular gorge was formed by the action of ancient glaciers, in this case, the overflow of a glacial lake. The beauty of upstate New York and northern Pennsylvania is captured in the view from the rim of the canyon. This is a land of farms and lakes where agriculture and tourism have always been the major drivers of the economy. The geology and the action of glaciers make this area special, but our geology also places us at a crossroads. Do we want to risk sacrificing this natural wonder for the temporary gain of extracting gas from far below, or do we find other energy sources that allow us to protect the land and water?

We are told that we can have it both ways. The experience of the Jameson family suggests otherwise.

As of July 2012, the Jamesons' cattle seemed to be back to normal, and sod was planted in the pasture to restore the hay fields. As he does every spring and summer, Charlie harvested his hay fields to provide feed for his cattle. It was then that he discovered that the staples used to lay the sod and the blasting wire left in the field contaminated his hay, rendering it useless. The drilling company, always the good neighbor, offered to buy the hay at half the going price. And those five additional wells that it planned to drill in the next few months? The company increased the size of the well pad to three acres and informed the Jamesons that the new plan is to drill a total of *ten* wells on their property. As of late 2013, however, Mary and Charlie have lost thousands of dollars and have yet to receive a dime in royalties. The only gas that has been extracted from their land has been vented to the atmosphere or flared off into oblivion.

SEVEN

SHARON AND WADE
Disrespect of Farmers and Farming

Although in the United States, as in most developed countries, the population has steadily moved away from rural areas in the last fifty years,[1] the fact remains that without farming we would have no food. But farming is a demanding and financially risky business that is subject to many external forces that can influence the farmer's bottom line. The oil and gas industry generally takes the position that the financial gains that farmers reap from leasing land for gas drilling can provide needed income with little or no impact on food production. The reality is far more complex and varied. Farmers tend to have independent streaks, which is completely contrary to leasing land to the fossil fuel industry. Once the land is leased, control is ceded to the company, so that the use of prime farmland may be compromised for years. Even in the best of circumstances, access roads and truck traffic can divide pastures and affect animal well-being. In more serious cases, leaks from wastewater impoundments, well blowouts, and faulty well casings can affect animal health and reproduction, calling into question the safety of our food supply. This is the story of one colorful, strong-willed beef cattle farmer who has experienced little financial gain and many serious consequences.

In the summer of 2012, I called Wade Davidson to schedule a meeting at his home and take a tour of his farm and neighborhood. His wife, Sharon, answered the phone; she was friendly but said that I would be speaking only to Wade when I arrived, and no one else. She was sick and tired of talking about drilling issues. Their eldest son, Wade Jr., who helped out on the farm, felt the same way, and she asked that I arrive after 2 p.m., to allow time for Wade Jr. to avoid me. She explained that her husband had been telling his story over and over again, but no one was listening. The last group of people who visited stayed longer than Wade said they would. When she had returned from work that evening, she went directly to her room, without stopping to say hello to her guests. She knew this was rude, but she couldn't bring herself to talk to them. Still, she asked about what I was doing and why.

After I explained what compelled me to speak with farmers about fracking, there was silence from the other end of the phone. Finally, I said, "OK, I hope to meet you when I come out."

"Yes," she said, "and I'll give you my two cents."

Wade Davidson was the first person I spoke with about the impacts of gas drilling on animal health. I called him on the afternoon before a Cornell Sage Chapel Christmas concert in December 2010, and thought that calling him three hours in advance would allow us plenty of time to talk, but I was wrong. It was clear after the first few minutes that Wade had plenty to tell me, too much for this one session. We would need many more hours on the phone, as well as face-to-face meetings, and I would need even more time to study his records and results—all this before I could begin to understand what precisely happened to him and his herd.

Wade was also the first person I spoke with whose problems revolved around shallow gas wells and not unconventional wells (horizontal drilling with high-volume hydraulic fracturing)—the type I had expected him to talk about. This isn't to say that there weren't any of these types of gas wells near the Davidsons—there were two within a half mile of their home—but it was the drilling of the two shallow wells on their property that caused them so much grief.

Ironically, Wade was the *only* person I spoke with whose water supply was definitively determined by the PADEP to be polluted by the gas company's drilling activities. This surprised me because this is the form of gas drilling—shallow well using low volumes of water and chemicals—that I thought was "safe" and problem-free. I would come to learn, after researching more cases like Wade's, that conventional wells, using lower volumes of chemicals, sand, and water, can have some of the same problems as the larger horizontal, hydraulically fractured wells, such as well casing failures and surface spills. The difference is largely one of scale, with the higher pressures and larger volumes of fracturing fluids and flowback causing proportionally larger problems.

And Wade was also the first person I had met who inherited an oil and gas lease (the surface and mineral rights had been leased by the previous owner)—something that he neither signed nor wanted. For Wade, this was the monkey on his back that refused to get off no matter hard he shook.

I started with a blank sheet of paper on a clipboard and simply asked, "What happened?" Wade had been expecting me to call, waiting to tell his story again. Almost two years had passed since he had lost ten of his eighteen calves, and I would come to learn that he had told this story countless times to reporters, to the PADEP, to the drilling company, to friends and neighbors, to anyone who would listen. Wade is the guy at the top of the mountain who sees the invaders advancing and starts screaming, but the people around him act deaf. No one listens. No one responds. Nothing changes. So he keeps screaming.

In southeastern Washington County, Pennsylvania, a stone farmhouse, built in 1796, hugs the hillside at the end of a long, steep, rutted road. The Davidsons have lived and farmed here since 1988, beginning with a couple of beef cows and working the farm when they weren't at their day jobs. Now that both are retired—Wade from truck driving and Sharon from working at the post office—they spend more time helping Wade Jr. maintain the farm. Wade owns nearly fifty-eight acres of land, the surface and mineral rights leased on all but seven acres, which is surrounded by leased land.

When I visited the Davidsons in 2012, I asked Wade if he was approached by landsmen to lease these last seven acres. He laughed and said, "Three times! 'We'll give you this, we'll give you this, we'll give you this.' They kept going up on it. And I said, 'Stay off my property!'" The seven-acre patch juts between two other parcels owned by neighbors and interrupts the path that would be used to drill horizontally from the neighbor's farm. I wondered aloud if the gas company were to come out again, wanting to drill a third well, what would he do? "I'd fight 'em!" he said. "They've ruined my property once. They're not gonna ruin it again."

Before Wade and I toured his farm, Sharon brought me into their dining room and carefully opened a top drawer. She showed me a faded black-and-white photo, undated and unlabeled, of a man in his sixties: gray beard and hair, chiseled face, high cheekbones, and piercing blue eyes. I expected her to say this man was Wade's father or grandfather, for the resemblance was striking. Instead she said it was a photo she recently found in the house while remodeling. She had no idea who it was, but assumed that it was a former owner of the house from the nineteenth century. For Sharon, finding this picture was a sign—to hold on to this house and land, to stay and fight for their right to have clean air and fresh water, to keep their cattle and their way of life.

Outside their home, in the back, sits a monstrous tank, round and wrapped in black plastic. It's what I first noticed on my tour of Wade's property—not the beautiful stonework on the side of the house or the scenery across the valley. It is this water buffalo, this thing that Wade and his family have been both lucky and cursed to receive.

"The water buffalo was always up by the barn, and Wade Junior would have to run two garden hoses from the buffalo to the tanks and old bathtubs in the cow pasture. In the winter, the hoses would freeze, making it harder to fill. After doing that for four years, we brought the buffalo down here, closer to the pasture." The buffalo holds two thousand gallons and must be filled every four days, but sometimes Wade has to wait five or more days to receive water. "I told the delivery man, 'What do you want me to do? Go up and have a meeting with my cows—tell 'em to wait 'til tomorrow to get a drink of water?'" When I asked why the water was delivered late, Wade opened his journals and read the entries:

> Snow, eighteen inches—out of power, no water.
> Run out.
> Refused to bring a load.
> Run out.
> Filling swimming pools.

I mused, "So swimming pools are more important than cows?"

Wade frowned and redirected my gaze to the pasture hillside. "See that black pipe?" he asked. "That's where the water used to run when it was up there." He pointed to a bush below the pipe where an eight-hundred-gallon tank used to sit and collect the spring water. "There was a pond on the other side of that tank. You can see where it was wet—the water used to run down to the field—all our extra water. There's no extra water here anymore."

As we walked to the site of the lower gas well, I stopped to admire the stonework on the farmhouse, recently repointed by Wade Jr. We crossed the driveway, where earlier, at the kitchen table, Sharon had described how in the wintertime the water pooled and froze after the buffalo was filled and the hoses were disconnected. We traversed a long, narrow barn, and halfway through, Wade stopped in front of a covered motorcycle. "This is what Sharon bought me—before the industry come here—for my sixtieth birthday."

I don't know motorcycles well enough to recognize that this is a Harley Fat Boy—shined up after a recent trek through Connecticut with Sharon riding behind. Wade has been motorcycling about as long as he's had a hand in farming, ever since high school. "Somebody said, 'You did that with the gas money.' Somebody said, 'You inherited your farm.' Me, Sharon, and Washington Federal Bank [paid for these things], and we paid 'em off early 'cause we both work!"

We continued through this barn, mostly full of tractors in various states of repair. As we crossed into the lower pasture, Wade described the locations of the five water wells drilled by the gas company after his original water well—located closer to his home—was declared contaminated by the PADEP. "Up above that swing set, they [the gas company] drilled the first water well. They drilled one near where that dump truck is: they didn't get no water. At the end of the garden, they drilled two more. That makes four. Then out at the end of these round bales, that's where they placed the fifth water well." A well, according to Wade, which produced water so salty his family couldn't drink it.

I first met Wade not at his house but at mine, when he had driven up to Ithaca to speak at a conference in June 2011. At this conference, landowners from intensively drilled areas across the country came to speak of their experiences. I had asked him to bring all of his records and reports, so that I could understand what had happened on his farm. With two gas wells, four sources of water, water well contamination, and a substantial loss of calves, his situation was very complex.

In addition to his environmental test results and official correspondence with the drilling company and the PADEP, Wade also shared photos of his beef cattle and farm. The cattle looked like Angus or Hereford—some completely black, others sienna red. I later learned that three breeds were represented in this herd: Limousin, Hereford, and Angus. In one of the photos, his Limousin bull, broadside and black amid golden heifers, seemed twice as large as the harem mingling near him. This was the bull Wade had described the first time I spoke to him, the one that occasionally escaped, only to be found munching grass in his front yard. This bull was easy to handle, had a great disposition, and was the best he ever had. But this bull had been exposed, along with the rest of the herd, to the drilling fluids that shot up like a geyser during a blow-out when the second gas well was drilled in 2008. Wade admitted that just a few days ago, he had reluctantly replaced this bull, because this was the first year, in more than twenty years of raising beef cattle, in which no calves were born.

Among the documents Wade showed me, I saw that in September 2007, he received a certified letter, return receipt requested, from the drilling company, informing him of the company's intent to drill gas wells on or near his property or water source. In that letter the driller stated, "We will, as in the past, take extended precautions to protect and preserve water sources surrounding the drilling sites." Stapled to this letter was another one, dated two years later, from the same drilling company. This letter referenced the lower gas well, the one closest to the house, and the original water well, and without explanation, advised Wade that the drilling company would no longer provide his family with drinking-water service.

So that I could understand what had happened in these two years, Wade showed me an official letter dated March 2008 from the PADEP to the drilling company. It was an order to replace or restore Wade's water supply, which the agency had determined was polluted by the drilling company's activities at the lower gas well site. The dates and events clearly show that both iron and manganese in Wade's well water had increased above the maximum contaminant levels since drilling had begun. Curiously, the letter failed to mention the two sources of water that Wade's herd depended on (a spring and a pond) and that neither of these sources had been tested before drilling began. It also neglected to state that both the original water well and the cattle spring, the main source for the cattle and farming, virtually disappeared soon after the original water well was contaminated.

None of the letters explained that there were five wells drilled in an effort to replace Wade's water supply, and that the fifth one produced water that while testing normal, was not being used by the Davidsons, because it tasted like salt water. But as no abnormalities were detected, the drilling company was no longer obligated to provide drinking water to this family. Most importantly, none of these letters could ever explain the stress Wade's family has endured since their water sources were lost.

At his kitchen table, before Wade and I walked his land, I asked if the drilling company attempted to remove his water buffalo when they stopped delivering drinking water. Sharon, who was standing next to him, moved closer and began massaging his shoulders; she did this several times during our conversation, but especially when we discussed water sources. At the time, Wade said, there was talk of removing the water buffalo, but a friend made several calls to Harrisburg on his behalf, and it has remained on Wade's property ever since.

I noticed that from the beginning of the interview, Sharon had been politely trying to leave the room. As she had warned me previously on the phone, she truly was uncomfortable talking about what had happened to their water and to their lives, but she was drawn back to comfort her husband. Before leaving, Sharon summarized how her life had changed since their water became contaminated. "When we lost our well water, we had to hook up the house spring [previously used only for bathing, laundry, flushing the toilet, etc.] to the tap water. We don't drink this water at all. I wash the vegetables in it, but then I rinse with bottled water, too. I cook with bottled water. We drink the bottled water. We live in the country. We've never had a water bill—just the electric bill for pumping the water." She paused, giving me time to take this in, to understand what it would be like to live in this way, day after day, and to wonder how much this would cost.

"We spent eight hundred dollars last year," she said, "on bottled water alone."

A nauseating odor—like turpentine or gasoline—greeted us as we approached the lower gas well, which was actively producing with a horsehead pump (a pumping unit that lifts liquid out of the well). Wade was not surprised by the smell. I pulled out my methane detector, calibrated it, and started moving it around the base of the well. A foot away from the base, it started buzzing, along where Wade believed the pipeline was laid. At the top of the condensate tank, the odor was strong and smelled like paint. I was feeling sick by now, so we moved on.

Ducking under the shorted-out electric fence surrounding the well site, we began walking along the access road created by the drilling company. Wade described how his farmland is harder to work and less productive since the drillers arrived. "You can see where the pit was [for residual drilling muds, fluids, and cuttings], where the ground drops down. I said, 'Where's all my topsoil?' It's all stones and stuff now." On site much of the time, Wade watched more than two hundred large trucks bring stones onto his property to make access roads, and he noted that precious little of the excess stones and brush were ever cleared away. So he asked the workers to clean up and place fencing around the well site to keep his herd out. When they didn't respond in a timely fashion, Wade wrapped the site in orange cyclone fencing. "Ha! They didn't like that!"

Besides the drilling company and the PADEP, I asked if anyone from a federal agency such as the EPA had been out to talk with him. His answer surprised me: "Just the attorney general's office. It was a criminal investigation."

"Against you?"

Wade nodded and explained how the events unfolded. When it was time for the drilling company to remove the drilling muds pit from the lower well site, Wade asked the company to take everything, including the liner, as he didn't want his pasture to become contaminated.

Despite his request, the muds and associated drill cuttings, fluids, and toxic chemicals were all eventually buried on Wade's property, and the liner was ripped out and placed on the side of the access road we were now walking on, to be hauled away. Because the liner was not removed quickly enough, it kept blowing onto his hayfield. Frustrated, and afraid that pieces of plastic would remain in his hayfield and eventually be eaten by his cattle, Wade placed the liner in the middle of the access road, to remind the drilling company to haul it away. For this he was arrested for blocking and dumping garbage on the access road. I didn't have to ask him if he would risk arrest and do this again, because I'm sure he would. But on the second well site, he didn't have a chance. He never saw the liner and suspects that the entire contents of the muds pit, including the liner, are now buried in his hayfield.

The access road wound uphill from the site, cutting across the pasture to the edge of the farm. When the drilling company finished the road, Sharon's response was, "Cows can't eat grass off that road, and we can't bale hay off that road." The sky darkened as we continued, and Wade asked me if I wanted to turn back—I had no protection from a thunderstorm except my clipboard, and Wade had none at all—but I declined. Wade thought the herd was on the upper pasture, near the second well site, and this might be my only chance to see them. As we walked, I thought more about Wade's cattle — this was their pasture, and now it had changed, the ground steeper, rocky, and uneven, with toxins buried in the soil.

We approached the entrance gate from the public road leading to the driller's access road. From here, the trucks from the drilling company turned right to head down to the lower well site or stayed straight to the upper well site. I asked Wade if the drilling company ever placed locks on the gate entrances to his well sites. "Well, they was gonna do that here," Wade said, "and I told 'em, 'You start locking my property up, you can stay off my property.'"

When the drilling company first came on Wade's land, a flimsy wire gate stood where the proper metal gate was now. "Five or six times," Wade said, "the neighbors called me at night and said, 'Hey, you got cows and horses on the road here.'" Wade suspected that metal gates weren't initially installed, because they might slow the truck drivers down. "When they did come back, I put a stake in the middle of the road, moved my dump truck up there, and said, 'I'm tired of chasin' animals.'" The drilling company responded by installing the metal gates.

Before heading up an even steeper incline to a second gate, I turned back to look at the road and imagined the trucks going back and forth, at first to build the road and well pads, then to drill and hydraulically fracture the wells. Because I know of herds that have been exposed to wastewater, I asked Wade about dumping, leakage, and spills on his property. He explained that in 2008, when wastewater was being removed from the impoundment, Sharon noticed that the back road, leading from their access road to the stop sign, was wet when she left for work at 6 a.m. "Just that road," Wade added. "After the stop sign, everything was dry." This was not surprising, as I've seen wastewater trucks in Pennsylvania driving with open valves on back roads, presumably to decrease the volume of the wastewater for disposal. Although spreading wastewater on roads is now legal under limited circumstances in Pennsylvania—to reduce dust and for deicing—it does require a permit and some minimal testing of the waste.

Further ahead, we saw some of the calves—white faces and red faces—born during the spring of 2012, but they saw us first and most bolted before I could get a good look. They were curious about me, but because of Wade's presence, I hoped to have a second chance. As we continued up a slope, Wade pointed to his pasture on the right. "This is where the wastewater pond [impoundment] was. You see how it's built up real high? I am leery of cutting hay here because of all the rocks left behind, and I don't know what's there."

Soon, the second well site came into view, and beyond that, a small pond that used to be a source of water for Wade's herd. There was no odor here, but at the base of the wellhead, the methane detector buzzed crazily, making the increase discovered at the first site seem small. I asked Wade if he knew about this leak—if anyone from the PADEP knew about it, or if it had been reported as a violation. He explained that no one had been out to inspect this wellhead, but that he was surprised there could be this much leakage as the well was only four years old.

Leaks such as this and those in pipelines throughout the country are rarely taken into consideration when comparing the greenhouse gas potential of using methane to other sources of energy, such as coal.

But just then—"Oh look, there's your herd," I whispered, so as not to scare the cattle. They had returned to get a closer look at what we were doing. According to Wade, they could sense when strangers were around and even knew when he dressed differently.

"And there's the bull—the red Angus," Wade said. "He's not as big as the black one [Wade's previous bull]; he's only two and a half years old. Not as nice as the black one, either."

This bull was big and beautiful. He exuded strength. Wade explained that you might find one bull in your lifetime with a good disposition, or you might not. The black bull had been one he trusted, and his son had trusted him too. "Wade Junior said he's leery about this one. You gotta watch him. He hasn't done anything wrong, but he's just not like that big black bull. OK, let's go under the fence, and I'll show you the pond."

Wade said this perhaps a bit too cavalierly, a bit too soon following his description of this red bull's behavior. The only thing separating me from this bull was an electric fence. But the pond was on the other side of this line, and Wade was carefully holding up the fence for me to roll under. The herd, including the bull, was less than fifty feet away. I believe you should never trust a bull, any bull, under any circumstances, but Wade was here, calm and confident, almost nonchalant, and I respected his opinion. I rolled. The herd moved off a little distance, just out of reach. The bull was not snorting or charging, was not acting any differently than the cows and calves.

Wade has a feeder calf operation, meaning he'll sell this year's crop of calves next spring, when they are approximately twelve months old. Some of his big cows are twelve to fourteen years old, and he keeps them around as long as they are throwing (producing) nice calves and they have good appetites. I asked how long he'll keep this new bull.

"I'll keep him ten to twelve years," he said. "The black one was only nine years old. There was nothing wrong with him except he wasn't making calves."

Wade, who happened to have been on the upper well site when the blow-out occurred, observed a muddy liquid shooting straight up from the well during drilling operations in early 2008. "When the geyser happened," he explained, as we now walked the path the drilling fluids took, "the muddy water ran under the fence and into the pasture and pond. The cows were walking through it and they were drinking it." This incident was not recorded by the PADEP as a violation, even though Wade reported it and has many photos depicting muddy water cutting through the snow from the well site to the cattle's pond—and showing the brownish tinge the pond soon developed. But by the end of 2013, no entry for this event can be found on the PADEP's website. Neither at the time of this occurrence nor at any time thereafter was Wade warned that the muddy fluid escaping from the well pad might have an effect on the health of his cattle. Instead, the health problems he observed in his herd were blamed on the "luck of the farmer" and *E. coli* contamination.

When I first spoke with Wade, in December 2010, what I heard on the other end of the line was a farmer who was very upset about losing so many calves, and if I didn't know better, I would have thought this was a recent loss, not one that took place over two years ago. As I would come to learn from Wade as well as his veterinarian, this loss was highly unusual: preceding drilling operations, he lost approximately one animal out of his herd of twenty every few years to illness or accident.

During the first calving season following the drilling of the two gas wells on Wade's property, ten out of eighteen bred cows, all of which had been exposed to drilling muds for several months either through pasture runoff or at the pond on the upper pasture, gave birth to dead calves or calves that died within twenty-four hours. Several of the calves also had cleft palate or eyes that appeared white or blue, or both problems; one calf was born with a nosebleed. A stillborn calf with white eyes is in the freezer, and the day I visited, Wade asked me if could I test it and tell him what had killed this calf.

I thought about the possible causes. Congenital defects (those present at the time of birth) such as what Wade's herd experienced are uncommon in cattle and may have an environmental or genetic cause. Because all of the calves had the same father, it's possible that several simultaneous spontaneous mutations in the bull's genes caused these problems, but this would have been exceedingly unlikely. If Wade kept his calves to breed back to the bull, this may have caused problems due to interbreeding, but as mentioned previously, Wade operates a feeder calf operation and sells all his calves each spring.

Environmental factors such as infectious or toxic agents could also be to blame and, like genetic causes, cannot be definitively ruled out without testing. Bacteria, such as *E. coli*, could cause septicemia in newborn calves, with cloudy eyes being an early sign of this disease. In these cases, calves either are born with the bacteria in their blood or develop the infection soon after birth. As Wade's calves were born with cloudy eyes, the only way for them to have acquired *E. coli* infection was in utero, either through the dam's blood or through an infected placenta. In Wade's case, the cows that gave birth to the stillborn calves were healthy with normal placentas, and none of the calves exhibited other signs associated with septicemia such as a swollen umbilical stump, pneumonia, enlarged joints, or diarrhea.[2] A virus such as bovine viral diarrhea could produce congenital defects, including the appearance of white eyes in newborn calves.[3] While this is possible because Wade had not routinely tested or vaccinated his herd, this scenario was unlikely because Wade's small herd was closed, meaning new animals were seldom introduced, and because Wade had operated with little to no calf losses for the past twenty years.

The last cause to rule out was toxic agents acting directly, such as the herd being exposed to chemicals during a spill, or indirectly, by suppressing the herd's immune systems and making the cattle more susceptible to infectious diseases. While difficult to prove, this scenario seemed the most likely because the only thing that did change on Wade's farm, after many years of healthy calf production, was the exposure of his cattle to the chemicals in drilling fluids. Ideally, Wade's calves should have had a necropsy to determine the exact cause of death, but that wasn't done. Would it be possible to do it now, two years later? I asked a veterinary toxicologist and pathologist, and both said the calf had been in the freezer too long. The next time it happened, they advised—send it in right away. For now, Wade has decided to hold on to the calf, to hold on to the only evidence he has.

In June 2008, after losing many calves, and after a two-year-old cow that drank from the pond died suddenly for no apparent reason, Wade permanently separated his cattle from their only source of water on the upper pasture. In February 2009, more than a year after Wade witnessed the geyser on the upper well site, his pond was finally tested by the PADEP. For a situation in which food animals were exposed to drilling chemicals, the test was remarkably scant, including only a few minerals, metals, basic chemistry parameters, and tests for coliform bacteria, including *E. coli*. Noticeably missing from the test were the organic compounds used in drilling fluids as surfactants, biocides, and scale inhibitors, some of which may cause both reproductive problems and endocrine disruption, such as 2-butoxyethanol.[4] Both iron and manganese tested high on the PADEP test of the cattle's pond. Was it simply a coincidence that these same substances were also found to be elevated postdrilling in the Davidsons' well water? No one offered an explanation for either the elevated iron and manganese levels or the failure to test for the other chemicals. Although the upper limit on the concentrations of these specific substances has not been established in water for livestock, it is important to note that because iron concentrations in drinking water greater than 0.3 ppm and manganese concentrations in drinking water greater than 0.05 ppm are considered indicators of poor water quality for people, they may also be a concern for beef cattle. In addition to iron and manganese, the fecal coliform count was also elevated, but the higher number was expected. Because the upper well site lies at a higher elevation than the pond, when the drilling fluids erupted, they ran across the pasture, taking along anything in their wake. Since the pasture was for cattle, manure was washed into the pond along with the drilling fluids, coliform bacteria (including *E. coli*) and all.

I asked Wade why the cattle spring and the pond—the cattle's sources of water—were not tested prior to drilling, as his family's water supply was. Wade had asked the PADEP this very same question a few years ago and was informed that these water sources weren't tested because they weren't for human consumption. "But I sell my cattle every year for human consumption," Wade had responded at the time, "and they drank this pond water for nearly six months before I fenced it off." And grazed this pasture for many more months, a pasture the cattle graze on to this day, a pasture where the soil was neither tested nor remediated. As would become all too commonplace, Wade's concerns were not addressed.

As we walked back along the edge of the pasture, Wade confirmed that in the second calving season postdrilling, five of nineteen cows failed to breed back (become pregnant), but those that did so produced normal calves. In the third calving season postdrilling, no calves were produced despite good health and normal behavior on the part of the bull and the cows. Consequently, as Wade told me earlier, he sold this bull at auction. I asked him about the fourth calving season, just ending now, and he said that eleven out of thirteen cows calved normally and that the remaining two cows failed to breed back. Before gas drilling operations moved onto his property, this sort of season would have disturbed him because it was rare to have anything go wrong. But for now, he was simply thankful for any calves to be born alive.

Crossing the next pasture, we found his horses—a quarter horse, an Appaloosa, and a Hanover—grazing. According to Wade, soon after the gas company placed new fencing on the lower pasture, his quarter horse ran into it, receiving numerous lacerations on his head and body. As he recalled what had happened, Wade's voice became loud and strident, and his body trembled. What upset him most was that this accident was preventable: the fencing should have been marked, and his horse, now covered with scars, could have avoided weeks of pain and healing.

Silent for a few minutes after telling this story, Wade regained his composure, and then apologized for becoming so upset. In his opinion, the industry doesn't understand farming or farmers. He said a drilling company in his neck of the woods is airing TV commercials promoting the idea that gas drilling can change the way farmers think about farming. "The gas industry says farming is for fun," he said. "It ain't got nothing to do with fun. It's work doing farming—raising your cattle and planting your grains and hays. It's not about putting gas wells on your farm—that has nothing to do with farming."

A few months after visiting Wade's farm, I traveled through Tioga County, New York, where a moratorium on horizontal high-volume gas drilling is still in place as of the end of 2013. I passed a big sign in front of a farmhouse: COMING SOON: NATURAL GAS AND MY NEW BARN. I think of these leased farmers, expecting to be happy. Perhaps they will be, if absolutely everything goes right. But even if everything is perfect, they probably won't be farming as many hours, won't be producing as many crops, and will have smaller herds because they simply won't have to work as hard. In the end, the question becomes not only one of the farmer's way of life or one of food safety, but where will we—as consumers—be buying our food if our farmland is producing more gas and less food?

Wade's case encompasses a number of important issues surrounding gas development on farmland. His cattle were exposed to drilling fluids and subsequently experienced reproductive problems; by the end of 2013, Wade's calf production is still below where it was before drilling began, and it seems he is caught in a vicious cycle, one from which his calf operation seems unable to recover. The health impacts of gas drilling were and continue to be a devastating financial blow that was not compensated for by the small royalties he was paid from the two wells on his farm.

And what about the beef cattle that were exposed and eventually went to slaughter on his farm or on others' with similar issues? Although meat produced in intensively drilled areas may or may not be safe for consumption, what percentage of cattle may have been exposed to drilling waste, and what are the long-term effects? At this point, we have no definitive answers to these questions.

Wade's case further touches on the issue of land use. Wade did not lease his land directly but rather purchased leased land, land that he never expected to be drilled, particularly since the lease was more than sixty years old when he purchased the property. When the drilling companies exercised their legal right to drill, the farm was divided by access roads, and the fencing was compromised. The portion of the land that was restored after the wells were put into production was restored in a way that was no longer suitable for hay production and grazing. Essentially, the drilling company permanently altered Wade's land.

Beyond these material changes, the bottom line for Wade and a number of other farmers with whom we have spoken is simply a matter of respect. If his right to farm and the integrity of his land had been respected, if his concerns for the health of his cattle and horses had been respected, if the loss of the water that supplied his house had been acknowledged and dealt with respectfully, his attitude toward all the problems he encountered would have been different. Instead, he has been arrested for protesting contaminated trash in his hayfield, is forced to purchase drinking water, and has lost more money than he's gained in royalties due to the devastation drilling has brought to his farm.

After all the work he has done on his house and land, I wondered if Wade would ever leave this farm. He said that he would move in a minute to a place that has good water, but only under one condition—that he could bring his cattle and horses with him. "If I can't take my animals with me," he said, "ain't no sense living. I'll go down dying right here, because I've got farming in my blood."

EIGHT

ENVIRONMENTAL JUSTICE

Environmental Justice is the fair treatment and meaningful involvement of all people regardless of race, color, national origin, or income with respect to the development, implementation, and enforcement of environmental laws, regulations, and policies. EPA has this goal for all communities and persons across this Nation. It will be achieved when everyone enjoys the same degree of protection from environmental and health hazards and equal access to the decision-making process to have a healthy environment in which to live, learn, and work.

—US Environmental Protection Agency[1]

NIMBY Not in my backyard. Anyone who brings up problems associated with gas drilling or suggests that shale gas extraction may not be the best idea since the Emancipation Proclamation is often referred to as a NIMBY. The argument is that if you use any sort of fossil fuel, then you had better be willing to have a drill pad next to your home. We recently checked Google Maps to locate the well pads near the home of the recently departed CEO of Chesapeake Energy and were unable to find them. A curious finding—perhaps the map was outdated. Although we have seen well pads near expensive homes in Pennsylvania, the areas that are intensively drilled are largely rural and not particularly prosperous. This leaves us with the question of who pays and who gains.

We are often presented with the positive economic aspects of shale gas extraction—more jobs and lower prices for natural gas. The reality, as always, is more complex. There is no doubt that jobs in the drilling industry have become available in the shale gas areas and that this has stimulated the hotel, fast-food, and trucking industries. Natural gas prices are down, in part due to the glut in the market. But understanding both sides of the equation, the benefits and the drawbacks, is key to assessing the impact of this industry.

This analysis should include both the long-term consequences and the uneven effects on different parts of society. A stock market bubble can benefit Wall Street investors, but have little or no effect on an elderly person with a fixed income. We cannot judge the health of the economy on the basis of the net worth of wealthy investors any more than we can judge the benefits of shale gas on the basis of temporary jobs created during the boom cycle.

Evaluating the impact of income to local and state governments—such as tax on gas extraction, multiplier effects associated with increased local business, donations to schools and hospitals—must be balanced by the costs of road repair, crime, health care, and massive tax subsidies, as well as the costs associated with the inevitable decline following the gas boom. The loss of traditional businesses such as tourism and agriculture also needs to be factored into the equation. When all factors are taken into consideration, neither the long-term nor the short-term economic benefits of shale gas extraction on local communities are evident.[2] And that is even before we begin to consider changes in traditional ways of life and other aspects of community disruption.

We discussed the idea of landowner rights in the previous chapters. The notion that landowners should be able to do whatever they like with their land, including allowing large-scale industrial gas drilling, presupposes that the effects are limited to the owners' properties. Yet it takes little more than a short visit to shale gas country to realize that when drilling arrives, the whole community is affected.

The notion that the decision to allow gas drilling into a community should be based mainly on the opinions and business practices—essentially the votes—of those owning the most land is profoundly antidemocratic. Since the 1964 Supreme Court decision in *Reynolds v. Sims*,[3] the law of the land has been one person, one vote, rather than one acre, one vote. Yet, a few large landowners can change the character of a community seemingly overnight. The question is really whether local governments can control land use or whether the state exempts local governments from control, effectively allowing the largest landowners to decide (by leasing) whether drilling will occur within the community.

In New York, for example, Article 23-0303 of the Environmental Conservation Law[4] stipulates that local governments cannot regulate oil and gas drilling. Some people have taken this part of the law to apply to local zoning—that is, zoning would be considered a type of regulation that is restricted under the law. However, New York State law considers zoning a land-use issue that is the purview of local government under the general principle of home rule. Thus far, the courts have ruled unanimously in favor of home rule, even after Norse Energy, a Norwegian company, appealed decisions to support the zoning laws in two small upstate communities that restrict the location of oil and gas wells.[5] The case went before the New York State Court of Appeals, and a decision is expected in the spring of 2014, despite the bankruptcy (Chapter 7 liquidation) of the US subsidiary of Norse Energy.[6]

In Pennsylvania, Act 13[7] was passed by the Republican-dominated legislature and signed into law by the Republican governor Tom Corbett in February 2012. Among a large number of other changes to oil and gas law, Act 13 removed the ability of local governments to apply zoning to the location of oil and gas wells. In July 2012, the Commonwealth Court found that this provision of Act 13 was unconstitutional,[8] and the case is now being appealed in late 2013. As of early 2014, local governments in both New York and Pennsylvania do have the right to restrict the location of gas drilling, but this may change at any time depending upon the whims of the higher courts.

Within a community, however, the issue of shale gas extraction is often highly contentious. This is illustrated dramatically in the plight of a small town in the Delaware Valley of New York. Sanford lies in the western portion of the Catskills not far from the Pennsylvania border. Some of the town officials reportedly have a financial stake in seeing drilling move forward in their area. On the other hand, considerable opposition to drilling is present in the town. The opponents urged the board to pass a ban on hydraulic fracturing, and the town board replied by passing a resolution urging the state to issue permits for shale gas extraction and banning further discussion of this issue during the public comment period of town board meetings. A First Amendment lawsuit was then filed against the town by the Natural Resources Defense Council and Catskill Citizens for Safe Energy. The town board ultimately backed down and rescinded the ban, and the lawsuit was dropped.[9]

Similar dramas are being played out throughout the Marcellus Shale region. This issue has inflamed tempers and pitted neighbor against neighbor. One of the most interesting aspects of this debate is that it cuts across political philosophies and is not a left-versus-right, red-versus-blue issue. We can point to both ardent environmentalists and Tea Party Republicans who are bitterly opposed to unconventional fossil fuel extraction,[10] and more moderate politicians who think that this process is the best thing that has ever happened for the environment.[11]

But irrespective of politics, unconventional fossil fuel extraction is a divisive issue in shale country, unlike anything else except maybe gun control legislation. Perhaps it is easy to see why. The debate involves people who believe that they will make a lot of money, and others who see their way of life disintegrating. But caught in the middle are the poor, with little or no prospects of making money from shale gas and little material wealth to protect themselves when their lives are shaken by drilling activities.

The rural poor do not have a seat at the table in any discussions of whether or where shale gas extraction should occur, even though drilling often tends to occur in areas that are not particularly prosperous— the land of the rural poor. While air and water pollution knows no socioeconomic bounds, dealing with pollution is a socioeconomic issue: the wealthy are better able to cope with pollution than are the poor. An investment banker living in a million-dollar home near a gas drilling operation can pay for a new source of water and install air filters, or simply pick up and move. A couple living from paycheck to paycheck or a widow scraping by on social security has few options other than to do without in order to afford to buy bottled water.

Proponents of gas drilling often argue that that if people think their water is contaminated, they can just use their royalty income to pay for water—problem solved. A flaw in that argument is that not everyone in shale gas country receives royalties, and pollution does not magically avoid those without a drilling lease. If you are receiving royalties, you can perhaps pay for a water buffalo or a lawyer to plead your case in court. But a poor family not receiving any income from drilling can afford neither a new water source nor the legal muscle to compel the township or drilling company to supply water.

We are going to end our series of illustrations on a bittersweet and inspiring note. This is the story of one family living in an intensively drilled area with stark contrasts between rich and poor. A subdivision with large, expensive homes is situated within a few miles of a relatively poor community. The subdivision has good roads, mail delivery, trash pickup, and, perhaps most importantly, newly laid water lines that will supplant the well water that the residents had previously used. Interestingly, construction of water lines carrying city water to the more prosperous areas of the shale gas regions of Pennsylvania rivals even the pipeline construction for natural gas. The nearby community that we visited has barely passable roads, no mail delivery, and no trash pickup. In fact, ambulances and fire trucks are reluctant to enter the community depending upon the weather. Most importantly, no water lines are being laid and the residents are forced to either use well water or come up with another solution for their water. The EPA's promise of environmental justice is not being fulfilled here. This community is not receiving "the same degree of protection from environmental and health hazards"; nor does it have "equal access to the decision-making process." The residents of the community are not empowered by society, but they are empowered to help each other.

The major problem in this community is that many of the homes have seen significant changes in the quality or quantity of their water, or both, since unconventional gas drilling began. We have made the point that drilling has pitted neighbor against neighbor. To some extent, that is true here. The people of this small community who have chosen to speak out about the water and air problems are not well received by nearby farmers with considerable royalty income. But within the small community, we experienced a different dynamic, one that provides hope and inspiration. These are people who have not been blessed with material wealth or political power, but who pull together day to day to help each other deal with the loss or contamination of their water supply.

NINE

CLAIRE AND JASON
Forsaken Community

Amid the dozens of people I'd visited in Pennsylvania to discuss gas drilling, Claire and Jason Wasserman stood out. I had expected that at least some of the people I'd be meeting would have signage on their lawns expressing their lack of support for fracking. So I was surprised that while driving through a large swath of Pennsylvania, where shale gas extraction is making its mark, I saw few signs of protest until I arrived at the Wassermans' residence. I'd seen plenty of signs, especially in Washington and Greene Counties, referring to the upcoming 2012 election and Obama's supposed "war on coal." The signs in front of the Wassermans' house reading "No Fracking" were not a surprise, as Claire had mentioned these as a landmark when I asked for directions. But it was so very striking that there were no other signs in this neighborhood where more than a third of the residents had been afflicted with poor water quality coincident with the arrival of shale gas operations. I was also surprised by the Wassermans' humble surroundings. Because Claire and Jason took the lead in organizing a water drive, and because they gave up their own water rations to neighbors who were running low and paid for some neighbors who couldn't otherwise afford water, I had expected that they would have more because they were giving more. But if anything, the opposite was true. While many of their neighbors seemed to be living at a similar level of sustenance, quite a few others lived in nicer abodes, had nicer cars and yards. These were my observations, not the Wassermans'. To them, these things were not important, were not discussed. The most important thing was water and helping others.

. . .

Claire and Jason are both from Butler County, just north of Pittsburgh.
They attended the same high school, Claire hailing from the country,
and Jason from the city. Their property, with its mineral rights leased
before they bought it, occupies 1.5 acres in a wooded community that
seemed to me from the outset to be isolated from other houses in the
area simply by the change in the surface of the roads. On the satellite
map, this community looked as if someone doodled a small square of
crosshatched lines onto a large canvas of hills, fields and forests, and
filled in the lines with side-by-side small boxes. The road leading into
the community was a very bumpy, narrow, unpaved lane, and I assumed
that the surface would change soon, for who could be expected to tolerate a road such as this day in and out? But this was not the case: another
turn, and I was onto the Wassermans' lane, surface unchanged. As I
discovered later when Claire graciously took me on a tour, all of the
roads threading throughout this small community were in the same terrible condition.

Over the few hours that I spent with the Wassermans, I would learn
that their community was segregated from the rest of the town regarding the services the people living here received: namely, in this small
wooded community of homes and trailers, garbage must be taken to the
entrance of the community, the roads go unplowed and unsalted in the
wintertime, and fire trucks and ambulances stop at the entrance, fearing
that they will get stuck. On several occasions, Jason has brought people
to the ambulance in his pickup truck.

For the past twenty years, Claire and Jason have lived in this community—Claire, a housewife, and Jason, a retired water-well driller de-
scended from generations of water-well drillers. When I first learned of
Jason's former occupation, I was excited to meet him. Here was someone who had expertise in drilling wells and could give me insight into
what was happening in his community. One of the first questions I asked
him in person was one that I'd had in mind for the past year, since the
summer of 2011, when I first spoke with the Wassermans by phone. At
that time, it had been more than six months since they stopped drinking
their well water, more than six months since purple suds and foam first
erupted out of their taps, and more than six months since both they and

their pets first became ill after drinking the water. I learned that soon after their water had become undrinkable, the drilling company had provided a water buffalo, and Jason had noted that the level of water in their water well was twenty feet higher than usual.

Now, a year later and meeting them in person, I asked him why he thought the water had risen so high. Before Jason could answer, Claire interrupted, "But some of the neighbors on this road—the wells have risen up to a hundred feet or more."

"That's because they are a different style of well," Jason answered. "The shallower wells will be a pounder, and the deeper ones—three to four hundred feet deep, they'll be rotary wells. We have a neighbor three roads over with a three-hundred-foot well. The water level was always at two hundred feet; now it's thirty feet from the top."

I understand that the levels in the water wells in this community rose after shale gas drilling began, but I want to know exactly what was it about this process that caused these levels to rise.

"They pumped four to seven million gallons of water per hole, and there are about thirty holes across that hill," Jason said, referring to nearby shale gas wells. "Basically, the aquifer was flooded. It blew out my hot-water tank. It blew out my pump." Jason believes that casings— several, an inch between each one, cemented off—were not used below one thousand feet, and shale gas wells typically reach five thousand to eight thousand feet in this area of Pennsylvania. "We are surrounded by old oil and gas wells," he said, "twenty-five hundred to thirty-five hundred of these. Plus old coal mines. Everything filled up after fracking."

Jason's well is approximately one hundred feet deep, and before unconventional drilling began in his area, the top level of water in his well was eighty feet down; now, the top level of water is at sixty feet. He asked me, "How do you raise an unlimited supply of water like that? There has to be a tremendous, absolutely tremendous amount of pressure. And a tremendous amount of water."

The Wassermans contacted the PADEP. Because Jason was a well driller by trade, and because he so intimately knew the water wells in his neighborhood, I assumed his complaints would be taken seriously. But both Jason and Claire have been disappointed by how the PADEP responded. They were left with the impression that they were the only

ones in their neighborhood with water problems and with illness associated with the water quality changes. Then people began knocking at
their door, asking, "What's going on here?" The Wassermans were surprised to learn that some of their neighbors had problems with their
water and were experiencing bloody noses and gastrointestinal problems too.

Before Claire described what happened to her family's health when their
water quality changed, I first learned what happened to their cats' and
dogs' health, in particular Rex, their beloved six-year-old Lab mix. On
the week of January 24, 2011, both Claire and Jason experienced digestive turmoil, projectile vomiting, and diarrhea. At first they thought it
was due to something they had eaten or a stomach virus. They continued to drink their water even though their two cats and three dogs refused to do so. But it was Rex who had the most severe symptoms—quickly,
he became very weak and unable to stand, began vomiting blood, and
died before Claire could bring him to her veterinarian.

At this time, another family who hauled water from the Wassermans' well (because it was ordinarily of such excellent quality) also became violently ill with vomiting and diarrhea. Yet both families kept
drinking the water until January 31, when Jason arose at two o'clock in
the morning to bring some water to his wife, and was shocked to see
purple-pink suds and foam coming out of the tap, filling up the sink.
Claire later recalled that the week before January 31, she had noticed
that plastic dishware left in the sink was turning a pink color that could
not be removed, and the water in the toilet bowl was pink.

After complaining to both the drilling company and the PADEP,
Claire and Jason received a water buffalo and bottled water. In the coming months, testing by the PADEP on the Wassermans' well water detected toluene, *tert*-butyl alcohol, acetone, 1,3,5-trimethylbenzene, and
chloromethane—all chemicals found in hydraulic fracturing fluid or
wastewater.[1]

Despite this finding, both the water buffalo and the bottled-water
deliveries were stopped several months later because an environmental
consulting firm hired by the drilling company concluded that the taste,

cloudiness, odor, staining, and oily film in the Wassermans' well water appeared to be common in their area, and these changes were not related to the drilling company's activities.

The Wassermans' situation, like many others, is complex because there is usually more than one event happening at a time. Not only are wells being drilled and hydraulically fractured, but processing plants are spewing particulates into the air, wells are being flared, and wastewater is being spread onto the roads or illegally dumped. A timeline, with all available drilling data and reported violations, environmental test reports, and changes to human and animal health, helps me to understand what might have happened and unveil potential exposures, especially in cases such as Claire and Jason's.

In the Wassermans' neighborhood, shale gas operations began in earnest in 2009 and continue to this day. By late 2013, there were approximately one hundred permitted shale gas wells within five miles of their home, approximately fifteen shale gas wells within one mile, and six shale gas wells approximately one-half mile away. The nearest wastewater impoundment is within one-half mile, and there are compressor stations and processing plants within a few miles of their home.

When I searched the PADEP records, I found a number of reported violations at several well pads within a mile of the Wassermans' home. During hydraulic fracturing of a well at the closest pad in November 2010, the equivalent of a forty-pound bag of bentonite drilling gel spewed out into an overlying stream and created a *frac-out hole* (a cavity caused when excessive pressure during hydraulic fracturing causes drilling fluids and muds to spill out onto the surface of the land being drilled). The inspection comment was dismissive: "There was no evidence that a spill had even occurred" and "there was no visible impact on aquatic life," even though the violation was resolved on the same day it occurred (indicating no further follow-up) and even though surface waters had apparently been contaminated. Should a spill of bentonite be taken so lightly? According to its material safety data sheet,[2] bentonite is an eye, skin, and respiratory tract irritant, and according to animal studies, it may also cause cancer.

Of even greater concern was a report of "defective, insufficient, or improperly cemented casing" of a nearby well in September 2010. When a well casing fails, aquifers face a double jeopardy: contamination may occur when the flow of drilling fluids and hydraulic fracturing chemicals are on their way down the bore hole, and again, when the chemicals, gas, and toxicants naturally occurring in the shale return to the surface. In November 2010, another nearby well was reported for "failure to properly store, transport, process or dispose of residual waste."

These occurrences may or may not have led to changes in the health of the families and the pets in this community—I knew too well that cause and effect were very difficult if not impossible to prove in these cases. And my timeline didn't start to yield any potential incidents of exposure until I studied a report written by an environmental consulting firm hired by the drilling company to investigate complaints at four domestic water wells in the Wassermans' neighborhood, including theirs. According to this report, hydraulic fracturing of two gas wells at the pad where the aforementioned casing failure had occurred was completed just two days before the families drinking the Wassermans' well water and Claire's dog Rex became severely ill.

Claire Wasserman's health has changed dramatically since unconventional drilling hit her part of Pennsylvania. Although currently in remission from leukemia, she first developed it soon after shale gas operations arrived, and months later, she was also diagnosed with grand mal seizures, renal failure, and hyperaldosteronism. Although none of these diagnoses were specifically associated with any known exposures, one incident stands out in her mind. In August 2011, after Claire noticed a metallic taste to her water and a black stain on her dishes, the drilling company and the PADEP ran more water tests. As these showed no obvious contamination, the Wassermans returned to drinking their well water. Coincidentally, Claire's white blood cells spiked and her leukemia returned. After that, the family stopped using their well water except to flush the toilet; Claire's leukemia went back into remission.

Regarding Jason's health, I knew he had suffered a sudden massive aneurysm in his nose and sinuses in April 2010 unlike anything he'd ever experienced before, but I didn't know the details of how or why it happened. "They were flaring a well over here, and this happened during a big flare." Claire explained. "It was ungodly hot when they were flaring that off. It was, like, ninety-eight degrees. We were coming down the road, and Jason said, 'Oh, my nose is bleeding.'"

Jason interrupted Claire. "You gotta understand—I'm outside all the time."

I recalled pulling into their driveway—Jason was tinkering in the yard. He had more exposure than Claire did to whatever was in the air, because Claire was inside most of the day.

Claire continued, "I said, 'Pull over.' We were in the car, right below where the well was being flared. We got it [the nosebleed] stopped and came home. The next morning, [after] he woke up, he was standing in the bathroom, and he said, 'Oh my God, Claire, come here.' Blood was just pouring out of his nose. I said, 'Hold it up here, hold it up here!'"

To demonstrate, Claire tilted her head back and pinched her nostrils. "When he was holding it like that, blood started coming out of his eyes. I said, 'Close your eyes, close your eyes!' and it started coming out of his ears. I thought, 'This is it . . .'"

Recalling this episode, Claire was distraught and on the verge of tears. In the emergency room, the doctor kept asking Jason if he had been exposed to chemicals, and Jason said he had not.

After much research, the Wassermans realized that the occurrence of Jason's major bleed during a flaring event was most likely not a coincidence. The process of flaring a gas well releases many chemicals into the air, including volatile organic compounds such as benzene, toluene, ethylbenzene, and xylenes (a group of compounds dubbed BTEX). In addition to affecting the neurological and respiratory systems, BTEX compounds can be toxic to blood cells, causing changes in, and the destruction of, red blood cells (anemia), white blood cells (leukopenia and leukemia), and platelets (thrombocytopenia).[3] Platelets are important in clotting, and when their numbers fall, bleeding is more likely.[4]

Nearly two years after Jason's exposure and after many more flarings and medical rechecks, the Wassermans' air was tested. A number of chemicals were detected, including benzene, toluene, carbon tetrachloride, and methylene chloride. As in most cases, their air was not tested before shale gas operations arrived in their neighborhood, so it is impossible to know the source of these contaminants. But Jason reminded me that he lives in the country, in a very rural area, and that these chemicals shouldn't be in the air he breathes—shouldn't even be on the radar. He shouldn't have to think about them, he said, and we shouldn't have to talk about them. There is anger in his voice. And I realize that I am angry, too.

During my meeting with the Wassermans, I noticed cases of gallon jugs and bottled water stacked halfway to the ceiling at one side of their small trailer. This water represents their ration from church donations—twenty gallons per week.

"For everything?" I asked, shocked that this could ever be enough for drinking, washing, and cooking. Later I learned that the Wassermans' allotment is low even by the American Red Cross Guide for Shelter Managers, which recommends five gallons of water per person per day for all uses.[5]

Claire pointed to her water allotment. "This is nothing," she said. "I deliver water every Monday to my neighborhood. Depending on your family's size, you may get an extra five gallons—we just don't have the donations to supply the demand." Claire redirected my gaze to a far corner of the trailer. "This is special water for the babies in the neighborhood. And those two boxes over there and the one on the bottom is distilled water for people who are on oxygen."

Claire explained that the jugs that I saw on the railing of her front porch as I entered are for washing today's dishes. "I get those from my mom and my brother—refilled at their house. And this side," she says, pointing to more jugs on the back porch, "are for bathing for today. They heat in the sun. At eleven a.m., noon, and one p.m., I rotate the jugs—the ones in the middle come out to the edge, so that we can take a shower. I mean, this is our life."

She says this almost apologetically, almost as if she were embarrassed, as if she should have to explain to anyone, least of all someone like me, who is not facing water loss, why they have to live like this. I imagine she said this because of the surprised look that was probably on

my face. But I am in awe of Claire and Jason's survival skills, for thinking, OK, let's use the heat from the sun so our shower won't be cold
(I later notice a camp shower in their bathroom). Let's keep the jugs
separated. Let's keep exact count for each day, because this is all the
water we have.

By March 2012, the drilling company removed all the water buffaloes from the Wassermans' neighbors, forcing this small, quiet community to ask for help. Claire led the water drive with the assistance of local
churches and organizations, even though she was being treated for leukemia, seizures, and renal failure. When I asked how she managed this,
she replied, "Somebody has to. They are hurting as much as I am." By
late 2013, thirty-six families were receiving water donations; when the
drive began in March 2012, only twelve families were receiving water. I
recalled an update from Claire in June 2012. At that time, a neighbor
had become very ill after drinking her well water; Claire brought her
bottled water and said that the woman was feeling better within twenty-
four hours.

But there is another motivation for Claire. "I'm becoming bitter
because they [the drilling company] did this to my community, and how
dare they? My community—if someone dies, we gather food or clothing
or vouchers. Fire—we do the same thing. That's our community. But
how dare they do this to us? How dare they cut off our water?"

Claire had remained calm throughout our discussion, but now was
outraged. "I was getting very angry, very bitter, and I channeled myself
into this water problem. A lot of people have asked me, 'Why do you do
it?' and 'How can you do it? You know, you're living without water
yourself.' I tell them, 'I wake up every morning thinking about water.
From my coffee in the morning, until sleep at night, every waking second of my day is consumed by water. But two hours a day, when I leave
my house, bringing water to my neighbors and listening to what they
have to say, it is so therapeutic."

I asked Claire if it's true what I read in her local newspaper, that she
not only distributes water but also pays for water for others when donations are low. "I got a call the other day from a neighbor in need of water," she said. "I just paid for it, and this neighbor said, 'Why didn't you

tell us?' I said, 'Because you wouldn't accept it from me. That's why I gave you a hug and walked away.' They know I'm sitting here without water. There are people in this community—if someone is out of water before water day, they give up their water for somebody else. That's just the way this community is. Unbelievable. We get beyond people helping other people. This is beyond that."

As Claire and I left her home to view shale gas operations in the neighborhood, Jason warned us to watch out for the tanker trucks because most have an associated chaser vehicle—an unmarked white pickup truck. According to Claire and Jason, both of them have been chased from public roads for stopping to look at nearby well pads—either by the neighbors who have leased their land or by drilling company workers. Although I have never experienced such harassment while touring drilling areas, others have told me that it's not uncommon to be chased off the side of the road for simply stopping to take photos or look at well sites.

Claire began the tour approximately 3.5 miles from her home—her plan was to start from this distance and work backward, showing me as many well pads and processing plants as possible. The roads were narrow and hilly, and as we left her community, she pointed to houses with water quality or quantity changes since drilling began. For these residents, this meant that either the water could not be used, there was a scarcity of water, or filters had to be changed much more often. Claire knew each home, each neighbor, because of her community's participation in an ongoing water study at a nearby university. Results so far indicated that more than a third of her neighbors have been affected.

Soon we arrived where Claire wanted to begin. She stopped abruptly, asking me to gaze into the distance. It was a postcard view of hills and valleys, but eventually I saw the well pads tiered in three locations at three levels: a few wells not far from where we sat in the car, several more behind these, and a few more on the hill—all in a line. Claire, constantly on guard, moved a little way up the road and around the corner, where there are more tiered wells, this time on both sides. She asked that I look quickly, take photos quickly; we had to move on so as not to arouse suspicion, to reduce the chances that we might be chased.

About ten minutes into this tour, Claire asked me, "How many have we come across?" A quick calculation gave me more than twenty gas wells on just a few roads. She slowed to an open area, and again there was a beautiful view of hillsides and valleys. She stopped the car and asked me if I saw the haze. "Isn't that fog?" I responded.

"No. It's constant. It never leaves, no matter the weather. You can drive to the next town, four miles over, and look back—and you'll see it clearly because it's not in the other towns around here."

Pulling into the driveway of a neighbor whose water has been affected, we triggered what sounded like a kennel full of barking dogs. The house was perched on a ridge, its property surrounded by large fields of pumpkins and squash. To the right and in the distance, there was a panoramic view of a massive L-shaped impoundment and a compressor station with many green condensate tanks. These were the two well pads closest to Claire, with six shale gas wells approximately one-half mile from her home. On these pads, a casing failure occurred at one well and drilling muds spilled into a creek at another well; both events occurred during hydraulic fracturing. To the left, an access road snaked to another pad within a mile and a half of Claire's home.

I wanted to stay longer and take more photos, but Claire began to cough and said she couldn't take it anymore: headaches and a burning throat come on quickly and severely limit her time outdoors. As we looped back toward her home, Claire braked suddenly again within a mile of her home. On the side of the road was a well pad with a large, unlined impoundment, its liner recently removed, Claire explained, as she drives by this way often and would have noticed it before. The liner lay crumpled just off the road, while large puddles of brownish water filled bulldozer tracks left in the mud at the base of the impoundment. The pad was guarded by three sets of four large brown tanks representing the twelve wells drilled at this site. The air here smelled as if we were enclosed in a sewer and seemed to worsen the longer we stayed. Directly across the street sat a house, and as we drove away, I wondered what it would be like to live there, to sleep there, to breathe there, day in and day out. I wondered how anyone could live there at all.

Fields of vegetable crops surrounded this well pad, along with other pads we passed as we continued on this road. Much of this land was leased, Claire said, and owned by farmers who sold their vegetables at a local market, some as organic. Soon, we stopped again: two large tanks of production water—fluid that returns with the gas after the first few weeks following hydraulic fracturing and during production— occupied the roadside. We were close enough to see that the cap on one of these tanks was open, allowing the volatile compounds to escape into the atmosphere. Here, corn is king, not only surrounding these tanks, but also on both sides of the pad access road. Was the corn absorbing these volatile compounds? Could there be residues of wastewater chemicals in the corn kernels? To the best of my knowledge, no one knew and no one was testing.

Besides well pads and fields of vegetables, the next most common things I observed in Claire's neighborhood were abandoned homes: no water, no sale. She stopped in front of a tidy little ranch with stonework, wraparound deck, garage, front yard, and backyard. "This guy thought he was getting a good deal," she said. "He bought this house, but it has no water."

"Didn't he check into the water situation before buying?" I asked.

"No, because he paid cash. He works inside the garage. The kids play outside. They can't do anything with the house. Isn't it beautiful?"

Claire slowed to a crawl as she pointed to houses on both sides of the road where well water has turned color or slows to a trickle within a minute of turning on the faucet. It was clear that the river running beneath this community—the aquifer—was disturbed coincident with the arrival of shale gas operations. It's not difficult to connect the dots—to believe that the millions of gallons of the chemical-sand-water mix pumped into the earth at very high pressure under this community could easily disrupt the flow of the aquifer these people depend on, the aquifer that feeds their water wells and provides them with drinking water. It's not difficult to believe that this disruption could have displaced substances in the abandoned oil and gas wells present in this neighborhood, causing contamination of water wells. And it's not difficult to believe that this disruption could have brought toxic substances from the shale or fracturing chemicals into the aquifer and into homes via casing failures, naturally occurring faults, or human-made fractures that extended too far. But as long as testing remains incomplete, as long as the exact chemicals being used are not known and not tested for in advance of their use, there is little hope of finding proof of a direct link, a connection between the devastation underground and that above the ground.

Just a mile from Claire's community, we took a detour. Large, gorgeous houses with big backyards and manicured lawns have also had problems with their well water, according to Claire. But recently, these homeowners were provided with the opportunity to have city water as an alternative to using their well water—a choice Claire's community, as of late 2013, does not yet have.

"Plain and simple, we just want water," Claire said. "We don't care about anything else. Our air is destroyed—there are no changes that are going to happen there. I don't really have anything against industry coming in and doing their thing. Everybody needs a living, everybody needs a job to do, but if you can't do it right or can't admit to doing it wrong, then something needs to change."

In the middle of quiet country lanes and farmland, a large gas processing plant appeared just off the road: it has much frontage but also extends back beyond view, into the depth of the valley. This one is similar to the plant I passed on the way to the Wassermans' home, with many towers and elongated tanks, with gates and guards and large signs warning visitors to stop and register before proceeding. This is where the impurities in the gas from the many wells in Claire's town will be removed—impurities such as non-methane hydrocarbons, carbon dioxide, hydrogen sulfide, nitrogen, helium, mercury, and radioactive gas, including radon. I took a photograph of the plant, and later, when I was reviewing the picture, I noticed a security guard in the photo taking a picture of me. It came as a bit of a surprise that the guard could have possibly considered me any sort of threat.

Claire stopped on the side of the road and motioned to the house across the street from this processing plant, explaining that she and Jason used to live here years ago. She said it was a nice house, with thirty-two acres. As large as this processing facility is, there are plans for it to extend even further into this otherwise gorgeous valley, where cornfields and hayfields now inhabit the land.

The processing plant was supposed to be the last thing I saw on this tour. As Claire drove, I watched the streak down the middle of the road, on the opposite lane. She mentioned this streak earlier, but here it was again, darker and more obvious. "When it rains, the whole road is soap bubbles. We saw a truck with the cap off. Just drip, drip, drip. I have a picture on my phone—it said 'brine water' [production water] on the truck. What's in brine water that would make it become soapy once wet?"

I told Claire that without testing, we couldn't know for sure, but whatever was dripping on the road probably changed the surface tension, like soap, so that foaming could occur easily. Because surfactants (substances that lower the surface tension of liquids) are the largest group of chemicals by weight in hydraulic fracturing fluid, there is a good chance that production water would contain these substances.

Claire was describing how she had passed well-pad access roads that were wet with puddles on bright sunny days, when seemingly on cue, we saw one. Claire shouted, "Caught 'em doing it—the whole road is wet!"

And apparently just finished. The tanker truck paused at the end of the access road ready to turn on to the public road we were driving on, the white pickup right behind it. Claire slowed down and pulled over to the side of the road, just a little way past the access road. But when the pickup didn't budge, she drove on, turning down a side road, just out of view. From this road, we saw the long row of mailboxes at the entrance to Claire's community, and we could also see the duck ponds across the street from the newly wet access road.

After waiting a few minutes, I got out and walked to the end of the road to see if the pickup had departed. Unluckily for us, it had, and Claire picked me up and raced to the scene of the crime, ordering me to "get a whiff." The August sun was hot and the day cloudless, yet from the public road, we could easily see that the gravel road was soaked with many large puddles filled with a cloudy white liquid. I asked where the road led and if it would be possible to see this well pad, the one closest to her. She was sure we could not. This was a private road—someone did live at the end of it, but it was also an access road to a shale gas pad, with a guard shack at its end.

It was not necessary for me to open the door and lean out of her car, for the odor enveloped both the car and us as we parked on the side of the public road. It was unlike anything I had ever smelled. The best description of the smell was a combination of a sewer and my college organic chemistry lab after a three-hour session. Whatever it was, it made Claire and me so nauseated that we departed less than a minute later, Claire holding a cloth with her favorite perfume close to her face to block the foul odor we had just exposed ourselves to.

This is how she survives, I thought. If I lived here, I'd be doing this too, and I hate perfume.

A few months after visiting the Wassermans, I mailed a check to Claire to purchase water for her community. I received a thank you letter from her church's reverend, who is organizing the water contributions. The letter sums up what I had learned on my visit to Jason and Claire's home—that vulnerable people in this community, as in many other communities across shale gas country, are in desperate need of clean freshwater for drinking, cooking, bathing, washing dishes, laundry, and tending their animals. In a later correspondence, the reverend explained that what began as a short-term solution has become a long-term project with no immediate end in sight. He thanked me again for my contributions and emphasized that donations will be needed to purchase water until a permanent solution can be found.[6]

WHERE DO WE GO FROM HERE?

As we have shown, proving that a toxic substance exists in the environment *and* is the cause of health problems can be extremely difficult. The question then becomes, how do we proceed?

One argument that we have tried to disprove throughout this book is the assertion that no case has been definitively proven to show a direct link between unconventional drilling and a health problem. We believe that the sudden deaths of farm animals following exposure to hydraulic fracturing fluid[1] provides a clear link between gas drilling operations and health impacts. Another somewhat more defensible but misleading claim, that hydraulic fracturing has never been proven to cause water or air contamination, is often used as a surrogate argument. When people make this argument, they tend to leave out all aspects of the process other than fracturing rock, ignoring issues like surface spills, faulty well casing, and hydrogen sulfide release, and focus only on hydraulic fracturing itself. Except for possible interactions with abandoned wells and fractures that reach back to the well bore, the process itself may be unlikely to cause contamination when the shale layers are a mile below the surface. But in shallower layers, such as wells in Wyoming, Alabama, and Alberta and wells planned for Ireland, Northern Ireland, and New York, the claim remains to be proven. When the entire process is factored in, as we have seen, water and air can indeed become contaminated, to the detriment of humans and animals.

We noted in the introduction that the precautionary principle would put the burden of proof for environmental harm strictly on the industry. Although the strict interpretation of this principle is arguably incoherent (that is, both inaction and action could produce some harm), as we discussed above, the alternative is equally untenable. That is, in the absence of strict proof of a link between drilling and health effects and environmental pollution, we simply ignore all possible cases of air and water contamination. The solution will undoubtedly require a careful assessment of risk and an equally careful assignment of the burden of proof.

The easiest way to think about a solution is to consider the process of drug approval by the FDA. To push a drug through to final approval, the pharmaceutical company must use carefully designed protocols and criteria to prove that the drug is safe. The burden of proof is not on the patient taking the drug; the burden lies on the company proposing the drug for approval. That is actually a somewhat more sophisticated re-statement of the precautionary principle. The drug is not assumed to be safe and efficacious until proven otherwise. Let's take this one step fur-ther before returning to gas drilling. Ibuprofen is generally considered a safe drug, although with known side effects. Now imagine that a com-pany wanted to propose a new drug with many of the same therapeutic actions, perhaps working in a similar way but on a slightly different range of targeted proteins in the body. Could the company claim that the long history with ibuprofen proves that this new drug is safe? Of course not, as has been painfully shown in the history of the drug Vioxx (rofecoxib).[2]

Returning from our analogy to gas drilling, we are told that gas drilling with hydraulic fracturing has been done for sixty years, with no proven cases of water contamination. This claim raises two issues in our analogy. First, we know that large-scale horizontal drilling with high-volume hydraulic fracturing is a massive industrial process that is differ-ent qualitatively and quantitatively from the small-scale, conventional drilling of the past—perhaps even more different than ibuprofen is from Vioxx. Second, where does the burden of proof lie? Do we assume now that the process is safe until the public or perhaps an academic lab can prove that it is unsafe? Careful standards must be put in place to ap-prove new procedures that have the potential to affect public health, and the burden of proof must lie with the oil and gas industry, just as it does with the pharmaceutical industry. As it now stands, the burden of proof lies, sadly, on the affected and those of us trying to make sense of what is going on.

There are many realistic solutions between the extremes of placing all the burden of proof on the public, on the one hand, and holding industry to irrational standards of proof, on the other. Among the commonsense, but elusive, reforms is mandatory full disclosure of all chemicals used in the drilling process, including proprietary chemicals, before drilling starts and in time for extensive predrilling testing of air and water. Public health concerns should trump any claim of propriety information. All water wells within a two-mile radius of the proposed well should be tested before drilling, and after drilling and hydraulic fracturing. The tests should be comprehensive (including all substances used in drilling and fracturing and those expected to return to the surface from the shale layers), conducted by an independent certified laboratory with a clearly documented chain of custody, and paid for by the drilling company. All results should be freely available to all interested parties, including physicians, who are currently under gag orders prohibiting them from sharing information, as is currently the law in several states, including Pennsylvania.

This policy would provide baseline information, but the interpretation of changes in air and water quality after drilling remains problematic. Proving that any changes in the air and water are due to drilling activity and that the concentrations present may be a health risk is difficult at best. In 1997, the Environmental Defense Fund published *Toxic Ignorance*, a white paper in which the organization argued that we know little about the risks of commonly used chemicals.[3] This is as true today as it was when the paper was released. In particular, we know little about how low doses of some chemicals can produce long-term health changes. The best examples are the endocrine-disrupting chemicals that are present among the chemicals used in the drilling industry and that work differently at low concentrations than at high concentrations. Add to this the problem we noted at the beginning of this section: we don't know all of the chemicals that may show up in water or air during and after drilling operations. This is a difficult problem with no clear solutions, but the burden of proof cannot lie solely on the backs of those most affected and those who can least afford an effective defense of their health and safety.

. . .

After traveling throughout Pennsylvania and meeting people affected by shale gas extraction and observing the environmental consequences of coal mining, we find it understandable that many people now question the continued use of fossil fuels for energy production. But what about renewables? Consider the cartoon image of the environmental extremist, who not only rejects fossil fuels, but also blames wind power for being too noisy and killing flocks of birds, and calls solar panels an unnecessary blight on the beauty of the landscape. We have never met such a person, and most reasonable individuals would agree that electricity and heating are good things. All of us clearly need energy to maintain our health and standard of living, but we need to think rationally about the choices we make in terms of both energy policy and how we live our lives. More importantly, can we continue to enjoy our lifestyle while knowing that, to some extent, it comes at the expense and the sacrifice of others? After having explored this sacrifice in previous chapters, we would like to consider our energy use from the perspective of both energy policy and everyday life.

The use of fossil fuels permeates our society and will be with us for many years to come. The questions that we face are whether it is necessary to transition away from fossil fuels, how fast we can do so, and what the costs will be. Considering first the necessity of fossil fuels, there are three important concerns. The first concern is examined in this book— that is, the effect of fossil fuel extraction on those living near gas and oil wells. The second concern is that because the supply of fossil fuels is finite, extraction methods become more and more expensive and environmentally risky as the supply diminishes. The third concern is the effect of fossil fuels on climate change. We often hear of the debate on the reality of anthropogenic climate change. This is a scientific debate only in the minds of those who receive scientific information solely from unreliable sources and those who use the perceived uncertainties for personal gain. The reality of climate change is not a significant debate in the scientific community; only the details are matters of debate.[4]

Anthropogenic climate change is real and must be considered in any rational debate on energy use. The use of natural gas as a substitute for other fossil fuels has been promoted as an answer to climate change.

This claim is based on one small difference between methane (the major component of natural gas) and other fossil fuels. In methane, each carbon atom bonds with four hydrogen atoms. In every other hydrocarbon fossil fuel, each carbon atom has two or three bonds with hydrogen atoms and the remainder with another carbon atom. Because the energy released for a carbon-hydrogen bond is greater than that for a carbon-carbon bond and each carbon atom produces one molecule of carbon dioxide when burned, methane releases more energy per carbon dioxide molecule produced than do other fossil fuels and is thus said to be a "cleaner" fuel. This does not take into consideration greenhouse gases released during the drilling, fracturing, or production phases, or leakage of methane during the distribution phase. Because methane has up to thirty-three times the global-warming potential of carbon dioxide over a hundred-year horizon,[5] leakage of methane is an important issue. Studies comparing the life cycle of methane with that of other fossil fuels disagree on whether natural gas is a cleaner fuel when leakages and other carbon emissions during production are considered.[6] The only certainties are that insufficient data are available on whether methane is truly cleaner than other fossil fuels and that not all pathways of methane leakage have been considered. In particular, little is known about the full extent of methane leakage in the distribution system. We can argue about which fossil fuel is the cleanest, but the fact remains that the only way to slow climate change is to transition to energy sources that are proven to have *much* smaller carbon footprints.

So how do we overcome the difficulties of the energy transition? The often-heard refrain is that renewable energies such as solar and wind are unsustainable because they can only survive with government subsidies. This argument may be valid in the short term, but only because the competition, that is, the fossil fuel industry, has been supported by government subsidies and compensation for the last 150 years.[7] Not the least of this support is the vast installed infrastructure for the distribution of fossil fuels, much of which was publically financed. Although there have been some efforts to rein in the power of the fossil fuel industry, such as the breakup of the Standard Oil monopoly in 1911, throughout much of its existence, the industry has enjoyed tax breaks, lax regulation, and outright contributions to its mission from federal, state, and local governments. The fact is that all energy sources receive government subsidies. When considering all the externalities (the cost of pollution, direct subsidies, etc.), the International Monetary Fund estimated that the sum of worldwide government subsidies to the oil and gas industry was on the order of $2.3 trillion for just the year 2011.[8] In the years between 1950 and 2010, the oil, gas, and coal industries have received 70 percent of the energy subsidies provided by the US government, with most of the remainder going to the nuclear and hydropower industries.[9]

Consider a few extreme illustrations of the disparate government treatment of fossil fuels and renewables, from the federal and local levels. On the federal level, the invasion of Iraq, which had little or no benefit yet enormous cost to the US taxpayer, can only be seen through the lens of protecting oil supplies for multinational corporations. Imagine invading Germany if the US supply of inverters for solar installations were threatened. Meanwhile, on the local level, the installation of solar arrays and windmills is tightly regulated. In some states, it can take years to acquire a permit for a wind farm. In Pennsylvania, for example, the state legislature and governor attempted to remove the right of local governments to employ zoning to regulate the use of land for oil and gas exploration (Act 13); this restriction on local governments' rights has now been at least temporarily reversed by the courts. In New York State, local control of land use for oil and gas exploration has been challenged in the courts (although by late 2013, local control had been consistently upheld),[10] yet wind and solar installations are carefully scrutinized and tightly controlled by local authorities.

If the playing field were level, then perhaps the transition to renewable energies could proceed without government subsidies, but in the current world, that is unlikely. Nancy Pfund and Ben Healey, in their paper "What Would Jefferson Do? The Historical Role of Federal Subsidies in Shaping America's Energy Future,"[11] estimated that for the first fifteen years of subsidies (considering direct subsidies corrected for inflation), the nuclear industry received an average of 8-fold larger subsidy and the oil and gas industry a 4.5-fold greater subsidy than renewable energies. They concluded that Thomas Jefferson would have done "what our country has always done—support emerging energy technologies—to drive innovation, create jobs, protect our environment, enhance our national security in a time of rapid change, and to further a distinctly American way of life in which resources once thought to be endless are replaced by ones that actually are."

But there remain several important obstacles, such as storage and distribution systems. The most difficult aspect of making the transition to renewable energy for electricity is that the sun does not always shine and the wind does not always blow. Other than batteries, effective storage systems are still under development, and the best existing solution is a better grid that distributes the load and renewable energy production intelligently over a wide area.[12] On the positive side, the greatest demand for energy from the grid typically corresponds to when the sun is shining, and the highest winds often occur when the solar resources are minimal. This solution can allow us to rely more heavily on renewables. In parts of Germany, 30 to 50 percent of the energy in the grid is from renewables at peak times (with an average contribution of 23.5 percent to electricity use in 2012).[13] But unfortunately, until better storage systems are available, a portion of US energy needs will be met with fossil-fuel-fired plants. The goal should be to reduce these nonrenewable energy sources as much as possible.

We have found that our own experiences with the impacts of gas drilling have had a profound influence on how we use and think about energy in our daily lives. Moving away from fossil fuels (including gas heaters, electricity from the grid, and petroleum in the car) can be done in two ways. By far the least expensive and most effective method is to use less energy. This is the low-hanging fruit that is easily harvested and can have a significant impact. The more expensive approach is to generate energy locally in a renewable manner. Everyone can participate in the first approach, and while the second is more difficult, it is also available to many people.

People can divide their direct energy needs into roughly three areas: electricity, heating, and transportation. By decreasing electricity use through lower-energy appliances, switchable power strips, and compact fluorescent and LED lighting, and by a concerted effort to turn off lights and appliances in our household, we have decreased our energy use by almost 50 percent. The remainder is now supplied by a modest grid-tied solar array (i.e., solar panels that supply electricity to our home and car and send any excess power to the electric utility grid). In our case, we will recoup our costs in about fifteen years. This required an up-front payment, but other alternatives are possible—for example, financing that arranges payments at approximately the cost of electricity.

Other options are springing up by grassroots efforts. For example, a community called Ecovillage[14] in Ithaca has installed a grid-tied fifty-kilowatt solar array that is shared by the residents and produces about half of their electricity needs. Likewise, in Bainbridge Island, Washington, a community project includes a seventy-one-kilowatt solar array financed by twenty-four area families.[15] These projects have been successful despite modest solar resources. Other communities are using bulk purchasing and negotiating with installers to provide lower-cost solar arrays to multiple households.[16] Electricity generated by solar arrays can only be widely adopted in areas with net metering. That is, energy produced by the solar array is fed to the grid, and excess production is sold to the utility. Many permutations exist. In the state of New York, residents can bank excess production for one year and use that to offset electrical use. After one year, the resident is compensated for the remaining excess at the wholesale rate, which is considerably lower than the retail value of the electricity.[17] The advantage of this arrangement is that the grid is used as storage system, and the more solar energy generated during peak-use hours (daytime), the less demand is placed on the grid. The downside is that residents are not encouraged to make more electricity than they use, as the compensation for making more electricity is minimal. More advanced schemes, such as that in use in Germany,[18] have led to much greater adoption of photovoltaic technology.

But this is only part of the equation. In colder climates, heating is an important part of energy use, and the traditional choices have been either fossil fuels or electrical resistance. At the point of use, both methods of heating can be very efficient, but the production and distribution of the energy (electricity, methane, propane) lead to significant losses and environmental degradation. Fortunately, better solutions can exceed the efficiencies of traditional methods and are compatible with a cleaner energy future. Of course, the first solution should always be better insulation and passive solar heating where possible. A house designed to the German Passivhaus standard[19] can require almost no supplemental heating or cooling in most climates. Taking it a step further, heat pumps can supply two to four times more energy than is taken from the grid or from solar arrays. The energy is moved either from the ground (ground-source heating, often mistakenly referred to as *geothermal heating*) or from the air (air-source heat pump) using the same principles used in refrigeration. This type of heat can be used in even very cold climates and is a perfect match for grid-tied solar arrays or wind energy. Alternatively, solar hot-water systems can be effective for heating domestic hot water and supplying some space-heating needs.

Finally, transportation may be one of the most difficult problems to solve, since our entire infrastructure is built around fossil fuels. Obviously, public transportation, ride sharing, and Internet commuting can help, but in many areas, private transportation is the only option. What's more, many people, of course, don't have the option of working from home. In terms of cost of operation after purchase, electric cars are by far superior but suffer from driving-range considerations and the pollution and carbon emissions generated by the electrical production. Nevertheless, in terms of carbon emissions, electric vehicles are better than gasoline-powered cars in all parts of the United States and better than hybrid vehicles (combined electric motor and gasoline-powered engine) in most states.[20] Hybrid vehicles remove the range anxiety and are, in some areas where electrical generation is largely from coal, more carbon-friendly than electric vehicles. In our household, we use an electric car (Mitsubishi iMIEV) powered by solar panels for local trips and a hybrid car (Prius) for longer-distance travel. The additional cost of the hybrid Prius over a similar gasoline-powered car (about $4,000 in our case) is easily recovered in gasoline savings in six or seven years. With dealer incentives, the iMIEV was about the same price as the Prius, but the purchase was also eligible for a federal tax credit. This made the car very affordable. The efficiency of the electric motor and the fact that it is charged in large part by solar energy make both the carbon footprint and the vehicle's operating cost extremely low. As a bonus, an electric motor easily outperforms standard four-cylinder gas engines on our steep, glacier-carved hills.

·   ·   ·

We have tried to present what we believe are serious health problems associated with fossil fuel extraction by illustrating recent cases from Pennsylvania. These are real people with real problems coping the best they can. But these are only a few illustrations of the problems that exist. They are by no means the only individuals that have dealt with the negative consequences of energy production, and we are continually learning about people whose lives have been affected. Our goal in writing this book is to call attention to these stories. We realize that in the short term, all of us will be to some extent dependent on fossil fuels, but we can do much better to ensure that when we enjoy a warm house or a warm meal, we are *not* doing so at the expense of our neighbor's health. Regulations clearly vary among the states and among different countries, but ironically, in the states that are arguably the origin of the oil and gas industries (Pennsylvania and New York, respectively), the current or proposed regulations are some of the least effective on the planet. They do nothing to protect public health and little to protect the environment and are largely written by the industry being regulated.

We can do better than this. We must elect politicians who will write and enforce better regulations. Most importantly, the agencies responsible for enforcement cannot be those charged with promoting mineral extraction. This dual mission sets up unnecessary conflicts of interest that are not in the public interest but are, sadly, the norm in most states. So, the solution is better regulations and better enforcement of unconventional fossil fuel extraction in the states that allow this process. In states such as New York, which by early 2014 still did not permit unconventional extraction, the process should be banned until it can be proven to be safe through health impact assessments and definitive animal and human health studies. Most importantly, wherever we live, all of us must move beyond fossil fuels to a renewable energy future.

A Primer on Gas Drilling

We have concentrated on the effects of drilling with hydraulic fracturing in unconventional tight shale formations, but have only hinted at the technical details. Here we will provide a short summary of the process and define some of the terms used throughout the book. The colloquial term that has permeated the media and web pages is *fracking*. In one sense, the choice of terms is unfortunate, because hydraulic, propane, or nitrogen fracturing (or "fracking") is only one part of the multitude of steps that go into extracting gas and oil from shale deposits. Also, fracking is sometimes used on a much smaller scale in conventional oil and gas drilling and other types of drilling such as water wells and geothermal wells. Nevertheless, in the public mind, the term *fracking* is synonymous with the whole process. In order to understand not just the fracturing step but the entire life cycle, we need to know exactly what lies beneath our feet and to understand the chemistry and engineering that go into extracting hydrocarbons.

Turning the clock back a few billion years, we see that the continents were much different than they are today; the world is continually being reshaped by continental drift. The large area that encompasses Quebec, New York, Pennsylvania, West Virginia, and parts of Ohio and Maryland was once a shallow sea.[1] The sea is long gone, but various types of sedimentary rock, including shale, remain. Because of the organic content of the shale layers, they became the source rock for oil and gas formation. What we mean by organic content is not what organic farmers grow, but rather what organic chemists study—molecules that contain carbon atoms. These range from methane (one carbon atom bonded to four hydrogen atoms) to longer-chain hydrocarbons (many carbon atoms linked to hydrogen atoms) found in gasoline and diesel fuel. As discussed in the epilogue, carbon atoms can make four bonds, so a linear string of carbon atoms (with single bonds) would have three hydrogen atoms attached on the ends (methyl groups) and two hydrogen atoms attached to the carbons in the middle (methylene groups). The smallest of this group, methane or natural gas, is a gas at room temperature and atmospheric pressure. Longer chains of carbon (butane, propane, etc.) can be stored as liquids under modest pressure, but will quickly evaporate if exposed to air at atmospheric pressure and room temperature. Methane requires very low temperatures (approximately –260 degrees Celsius) or high pressures to be stored as a liquid. The shale layers trap these compounds along with all the salt that was in the ocean. The layers also trap bacteria, archaea, more complex organic compounds such as benzene, heavy metals, and radioactive material.

Geologists have known about the presence of oil and gas in shale layers for a long time, but extraction of these hydrocarbons for use as fuels originally did not involve going to the source. Instead, the traditional method was to find a pocket of gas or oil that was trapped underground. Although the shale layers are the source of the hydrocarbons, the gas or oil can gradually migrate upward over millions of years into layers of more porous rock, where it can get trapped under a layer of impervious rock. By drilling down into this pocket of gas or oil, the hydrocarbon can be extracted, maybe even with a little stimulation by low-volume hydraulic fracturing. The overwhelming majority of gas and oil wells drilled worldwide have used this relatively simple idea, which the industry calls *conventional drilling*.

Despite the vast amount of oil and gas that has been extracted from the ground over the last 150 years, the pools of gas are limited. Consequently, drillers have, over the last 15 years or so, employed more extreme methods to extract fossil fuels. The two methods that are the most controversial are tar sands (also known as oil sands) extraction and horizontal drilling with high-volume hydraulic fracturing. The environmental impact of the tar sands method is beyond the scope of this book, but has been carefully covered by Andrew Nikiforuk in his book *Tar Sands*.[2] We are concerned with the latter method, horizontal drilling and high-volume hydraulic fracturing (or propane or nitrogen fracturing).

The shale layers primarily discussed in this book are the Marcellus and Utica Shales in the Northeastern United States. The Marcellus is the better known and younger of the two—on the order of 380 million years old. It underlies much of the Appalachian basin, extending from New Jersey and Virginia through parts of Maryland, West Virginia, Ohio, Pennsylvania, and New York. It reaches the surface near the top of the Finger Lakes in upstate New York and is named after the town of Marcellus, just west of Syracuse, where it outcrops at the surface.[3] Although the formation is large, the area that is considered the best to develop is somewhat smaller, encompassing parts of West Virginia, about half of Pennsylvania, and the southernmost part of upstate New York. This is the "fairway," where the portions of the shale may be sufficiently deep and thick to make extraction of large quantities of hydrocarbons possible.[4] The Utica Shale (named after the outcropping in Utica, New York) extends over a somewhat larger area, under the Great Lakes, and into Canada.[5] It is older (more than 400 million years old) and deeper, but has not been explored as well as the Marcellus.

In both the Utica and the Marcellus Shales, the composition of the hydrocarbons differs in different locations.[6] For example, in northeastern Pennsylvania, largely "dry gas" is extracted from the Marcellus Shale. Dry gas is mostly methane, which as we have noted is a gas at room temperature and atmospheric pressure. As you move to southwestern Pennsylvania, more "wet gas" is extracted. Wet gas includes the longer-chain molecules, such as propane and butane, which are volatile liquids at moderate pressures. The wet gases are more valuable because they can be converted to other useful compounds in chemical plants or in petroleum refineries. These plants can convert, for example, ethane into ethylene (two carbon atoms bound by a double bond, with two hydrogen atoms on each carbon atom) and subsequently into plastics and other chemicals. The western part of the Utica Shale, particularly in Ohio, has become of great interest to the industry because it has begun to yield even longer-chain hydrocarbons, in the form of crude oil ("tight oil"). Oil is a more valuable commodity than natural gas.[7] Typically, methane is also present with the oil and is often just discarded as a by-product. That is, the gas can either be vented to the atmosphere or be burned in a dramatic manner known as flaring. A good example of this is the oil boom in North Dakota (Bakken Shale), where large quantities of natural gas are extracted with the oil, but because few pipelines are present, the gas is largely wasted by flaring.[8] This practice, of course, wastes the resources owned by private landowners, and a lawsuit seeking to recover lost royalties has recently been filed against several large fossil fuel companies.[9]

The Northeastern United States is no stranger to oil and gas extraction, as we mentioned in a previous chapter. In fact, one could argue that the oil and gas industries were born in Pennsylvania and New York. However, by going to the source, that is, to the shale layers themselves, the whole strategy used by the industry changes along with an increased impact on the landscape. In the past, small wells were drilled wherever pockets of gas or oil were detected. For example, driving around the countryside near the home of the famous Pennsylvania groundhog, Punxsutawney Phil, you can see older gas wells everywhere, and they are still in production. These wells were drilled into pockets of natural gas, which were common in the area.

Targeting the source rock means that huge areas of West Virginia, Pennsylvania, and New York can be exhaustively drilled with horizontal drilling and hydraulic fracturing. Proponents of such unconventional extraction will note that for a single installation, much larger areas can be drained because multiple wells can be placed on a single pad and drilled in all directions (or, more precisely, in a rectangular pattern). But the fact remains that much larger areas are now being targeted for production than would ever be considered by traditional methods. Given that even in intensively drilled parts of Pennsylvania and West Virginia, only a small fraction of the planned wells are in place, the environmental and societal consequences that we see now are only the beginning.

. . .

Let's narrow our focus and look at an individual well pad. The whole process starts with leasing land. A company comes into an area, and the landsman convinces landowners to sign a lease. The lease can contain surface rights, in which case the drilling pad can be placed on the property, or the lease might include only mineral rights, in which case the oil or gas can be taken from under the surface of the property. In some cases, the owner of the surface rights may not be the same person as the owner of the mineral rights. This might happen if the owner of a parcel of land leases mineral rights to a company and then sells the property (the surface) without transferring the lease to the new owner. Once signed, the lease can be bought and sold many times by different companies.

Before drilling starts, the site is often mapped using seismic testing. This is done either with large thumper trucks or helicopters and explosive charges. The idea is to provide a three-dimensional map of the geology of the area and to identify faults or other problems that might affect the efficiency of hydrocarbon extraction or cause environmental problems.

The drilling starts with the choice of a site and the construction of access roads. The site is usually five to seven acres of leveled land, typically on a plateau, the location of which is chosen mainly by the drilling company. Large ponds may be constructed nearby to hold millions of gallons of water (either water that will be used to hydraulically fracture the well or wastewater that returns to the surface). We have seen pads very close to barns and access roads that were within a few feet of homes.

Once the drilling pad is built, things can but do not always proceed rapidly, depending on the economic climate. As one strategy, companies establish wells throughout an area, perhaps drilling only one well per pad. Most leases are written such that once activity related to drilling begins, the lease cannot be canceled, so that establishing a well locks in the lease indefinitely. In any event, the next step is to drill one or more wells. This is when the iconic drilling rig is set up, and drilling begins. This is not your common, everyday well-drilling operation but rather an impressive industrial operation with very high-tech engineering.

The drilling company often uses three different drilling rigs in sequence. The first rig drills down below the water table, then a second rig that can handle high pressure if pockets of gas are encountered is put into action. Finally, a third rig drills the horizontal part of the well. The first stage of drilling is typically lubricated largely with air to help avoid contaminating an aquifer with drilling fluids. However, surfactants, some of which contain 2-butoxyethanol, are used in this stage and can be introduced into an aquifer. The drill bits for the second and third stages of drilling are lubricated with drilling fluids and muds.

It is this feat of horizontal drilling that really opened up the source rock for exploitation. Drilling vertically into a shale formation only allows the driller to contact a region equal to the thickness of the formation (perhaps fifty to two hundred feet). That is, since the formation is only fifty to two hundred feet thick, a vertical well can only make contact with the relatively small surface area surrounding the well. By turning the bit horizontally, the horizontal part of the well is in continual contact with the formation, and these *laterals* run long distances, typically about a mile and sometimes up to two miles, all within the shale formation. Thus, horizontal drilling allows a much larger area to be drained from a single well. By running multiple wells in a pitchfork pattern in two directions, a driller can drain a large rectangle.

But at this point, we have just described drilling a hole in the ground—a high-tech hole, but just a hole. The next issue to consider is the attempt to protect the aquifer with a steel and cement casing so that fluid can be injected into the well and so that gas and liquid can exit the well without contaminating the water supply. Several layers of casing are put into place surrounding the well bore to a depth well below the aquifers in the region. This is typically done after drilling the first stage. Failure of the cement around the steel casing pipe is one of the most common causes of aquifer contamination. Also, the cement does not necessarily make a complete seal with the surrounding rock and soil, leaving potential migration paths for methane that is released from the shale layers or more superficial layers.

The next step is to fracture the rock to release methane. The most common method is hydraulic fracturing, a process by which approximately five million gallons of fluid and large quantities of silica sand are injected into the well under high pressure (thousands of pounds per square inch, depending on the depth and pressure in the shale). (The alternatives to hydraulic fracturing are currently high-pressure propane and nitrogen fracturing. These are less well tested and may or may not be used extensively in the future. Propane fracturing carries with it the danger of explosion from accidents on the surface.) The high pressure fractures the rock, and the silica props open the fractures so that they don't reseal. In this way, gas can flow out of the formation. The fluid is mainly water, but contains many chemicals, including biocides (to kill bacteria), friction reducers, oxygen scavengers, acids, chemical cross-linkers, and scale and corrosion inhibitors. It is this hydraulic fracturing fluid that has probably sparked the most controversy and alarm. The major points of contention include the composition of the fluid, its toxicity, interactions between the components, how the components change due to chemical reactions within the well, and whether the fluid can contaminate the water or air.

Some chemicals in the fluid are known and are listed on industry websites such as fracfocus.org and the sites of individual companies. However, a major problem is that the exact composition of the fluid is not known *prior to drilling* by individuals who might be affected, negating their ability to test their well and surface water completely *before* drilling begins. Learning the composition of the fluid after the fact (e.g., on the FracFocus website) is of more limited value because it is impossible to prove that a chemical detected after drilling was absent before the drilling began. Moreover, the information released to the public is largely at the discretion of the company; proprietary information is withheld. The importance of this selective release of information is often downplayed, but a glance at the Material Safety Data Sheets of drilling components clearly shows that quite a bit of information can be withheld. Legitimate questions to ask state regulatory agencies are whether a company should have the right to withhold the identity of chemicals that might end up in our drinking water or our food supply, or that medical personnel might need to know about to safely treat people or animals exposed to the chemicals in accidents.

We often hear that the composition of hydraulic fracturing fluid contains 99 percent or more water and sand and less than 1 or 2 percent other chemicals.[10] Not only that, but we are told many of the chemicals are found in food and pharmaceuticals, so no need to worry. A public relations executive might think that providing this anodyne to the public would calm any fears. In truth, this information is sadly misleading and contributes to mistrust of the industry among much of the public.

Consider what is being said. First of all, sand sounds fine because our kids play in sandboxes and we all love sandy beaches. But this isn't your average sand. In fact, these huge quantities of silica sand increase exposure to respirable crystalline silica dust, which is a public health threat to the communities in Wisconsin and Minnesota, where the sand is mined. Furthermore, the huge volume of silica used in hydraulic fracturing operations is a major threat to the rig workers and to residents in communities where sand is stored on its way to drilling sites. Breathing these silicates is a well-known cause of silicosis, which results in inflammation and lesions in the upper lobes of the lungs.

The next question is the implication that 1 or 2 percent is somehow insignificant. In the biological and medical sciences, a 1 percent solution is often an enormous concentration that can be extremely toxic. In that sense, the assertion that the fluid contains "only" 1 percent chemicals is not reassuring. Also, 1 percent of five million gallons is fifty thousand gallons, which is not a small volume of toxic fluid.

The notion that the components are found in everyday products is perhaps the most misleading. The public is told that ethylene glycol is found in many everyday products and that glutaraldehyde is used to sterilize medical equipment. What we aren't told is that these highly toxic compounds should never be found in drinking water. Hydrochloric acid is used, and since it is a component of your stomach, it most certainly must be safe. But it is a strong acid; spills of hydrochloric acid have caused environmental damage and sent workers to the hospital in Pennsylvania.

The final question is whether this potentially dangerous solution of hydraulic fracturing fluid can ever come in contact with drinking or surface water. The answer all depends upon how the question is asked. There is little doubt that individual chemicals or the mixed fracturing fluid has been released into the environment, either through spillage on the surface or from the blowout of wells during fracturing. Fracturing fluids have been released into the environment multiple times in Pennsylvania, and each event is always immediately dismissed as unimportant ("only a few frogs were killed").[11]

The harder part of the drinking-water question is whether hydraulic fracturing—that is, the fractures—can contaminate aquifers. The argument is often made that contact is totally impossible, because the horizontal portion of the well bore is a mile below the aquifer. Industry estimates suggest that rare fractures can occur up to two thousand feet from the horizontal well bore, although most are much smaller.[12] Nevertheless, because hydraulic fracturing has been done in formations as shallow as two thousand feet (in Wyoming and Canada) and many shale plays slated for drilling are less than three thousand feet deep (e.g., in the Marcellus in New York; in Fermanagh in Northern Ireland; and in Letrim in Ireland), direct contamination of the aquifer becomes a greater probability. What's more, abandoned wells, if contacted by a fracture, can form a conduit to the surface or to an aquifer.[13] For this reason, abandoned wells should be identified by seismic testing, but they have been missed in the past.[14] Finally, natural fractures in the rock could be a conduit to aquifers,[15] particularly during the drilling of shallow formations. Thus, legitimate questions remain about the safety of the actual process of hydraulic fracturing.

After the hydraulic fracturing or fracturing with propane or nitrogen is done, the pressure is released and fluid and gas now come back up the well bore to the surface. The pressure deep below the earth's surface is high, so that the general flow is in the direction of the surface. In dry-gas areas, the drillers are seeking methane, so the gas is collected and the remainder is waste. In wet-gas or tight-oil regions, the methane gas and petroleum liquids have to be separated from the other liquids returning to the surface. Aside from the processing, wastewater may be the biggest environmental threat that arises.

Even when propane or nitrogen fracturing is used, wastewater returns to the surface in large quantities and has to be disposed of or reused. Before either of these steps, the wastewater is generally stored on site either in large lagoons (wastewater impoundments) or in metal containers. The leakage of these wastewater impoundments has contaminated soil and drinking water for both humans and animals, and wildlife (particularly birds) can be directly exposed. The wastewater is being recycled more often now than in the past—an approach with many advantages. It reduces the volume of wastewater that has to be discarded and reduces the amount of freshwater that has to be used. On the other hand, the fluid becomes progressively more toxic as it is used in subsequent wells, and while smaller in volume, it does present more of a disposal problem.

Disposal of wastewater presents another challenge. This step requires the removal of the fluid from the site either by pipelines or by truck. Leaks and spills can occur, introducing the wastewater into the environment, with the possibility of contaminating drinking-water aquifers. In our experience, at least some of the leakage from trucks has apparently been intentional. The wastewater can be taken to a water-treatment plant. In the past, treatment plants incapable of treating these fluids have accepted wastewater and released contaminated fluid into drinking-water supplies. An example is the contamination of the Monongahela River, which supplies some of the drinking water to Pittsburgh, in 2009.[16] More-sophisticated water-treatment facilities exist, but the safety of the process cannot be verified if the effluent isn't fully tested, as is almost always the case. For example, a recent study showed that treated effluent from a water-treatment facility that was processing drilling wastewater contained above-background levels of bromide, chloride, and radium-226.[17] Another use of the wastewater is for dust control or the deicing of roads, a process with the Orwellian name of "beneficial use." In principle, wastewater cannot be used unless tested for a few select chemicals. In practice, the testing is minimal and the changes in the composition of the fluid in different stages of extraction make the testing at best problematic.

Finally, wastewater is often injected deep into the ground. Although this method of disposal has been widely used, it has, in some cases, resulted in earthquakes. The events are not on the magnitude of the 2011 earthquake in Japan, but have measured 3 or 4 on the Richter scale. Earthquakes of this magnitude are rarely deadly but can cause damage. However, a magnitude 5.7 quake in Prague, Oklahoma, in November 2011 destroyed fourteen homes and has been linked to wastewater injection wells.[18] In 2012, scientists from the US Geological Survey found that the frequency of magnitude 3 or greater earthquakes in the midcontinent of the United States in the decade starting in 2001 was six times greater than the frequency during all of the twentieth century and that this was almost certainly due to human causes.[19] This increase in midcontinent earthquakes is the source of the often-repeated notion that hydraulic fracturing causes earthquakes. It is actually the injection wells that have been the cause of earthquakes rather than the wells used to extract oil and gas. And while the eastern United States is seismically active, it is nowhere near as active as California. With proposals to extract oil and gas in California using hydraulic fracturing and the necessity of disposing of wastewater,[20] issues of seismicity will undoubtedly be given considerable attention in the near future.

In addition to what happens at the well site and with the disposal of wastewater, the community impacts are important considerations. The public is often treated to the canard that drilling and hydraulic fracturing only takes a month or so at most and, after that, there is just a pipe in the ground from which riches flow. For a small part of the process, there may be a small kernel of truth in this statement, but overall, the idea is misleading. Drilling rigs are expensive, so the drilling time is indeed held to a minimum, and hydraulic fracturing, which can occur within days or months after drilling, may take less than a week to complete. But this happens only after the well site has been prepared and the access road built. Furthermore, additional wells can be drilled on the site at any time after the first well is drilled, and wells can be flared or fractured multiple times. In addition, pipelines have to be built to take the gas away and sometimes to remove the wastewater. All this heavy equipment and huge quantities of fluid and sand arrive at the well by truck, necessitating thousands of truck trips per well, often on roads ill equipped to handle anything more than the occasional farm truck. It is not uncommon for activity at a well pad to stretch on for more than a year or longer. We know of cases where activity on the same well pad has extended on and off for longer than four years.

Multiple wells are drilled to maximize the profits from drilling in a given area and to support the cost of constructing pipelines and other infrastructure. Living in an area that is intensively drilled is not a minor disruption for a month and then easy street; the people interviewed throughout this book have described it as an "invading army." While activity on one well may not be continual, from the perspective of the community as a whole, activity is indeed continual and disrupting. Multiple wells are drilled, hydraulically fractured, and flared; pipelines are built; compressor stations and processing plants are constructed; and the truck traffic is never ending.

This massive activity is a blessing for some and a curse for others. Indeed, some businesses thrive (fast-food restaurants, hotels, bars, nightclubs, gas stations), while others are disrupted (tourism, recreation [hunting, fishing, and boating], farming, wine-making, cheese-making, beer-making, real estate sales, bed and breakfast reservations, cottage rentals). Although the economic impact is often presented as positive, several studies, especially the work of Deborah Rogers[21] and Janette Barth,[22] have questioned this conclusion and have looked at both the positive and the negative drivers of the economy. Clearly, some people do see the riches, but what is the overall effect on the community, state, and nation? We cannot just consider the bottom line of multinational companies and the restaurant owner; the final analysis includes such far-reaching effects as water and air pollution, global warming potential of different forms of energy, and the cost-benefit analysis of switching more rapidly to renewable energy. But a switch to renewable energy will eventually be required, since fossil fuels are finite and extraction methods to eke out the last dregs of fuel on the planet will become increasingly more expensive and hazardous. The sooner and more aggressively we move to a clean-energy future, the better life will be for our children and grandchildren.

Weeks from our book deadline, one of us (MB) noticed an article in the *New York Times*, "Two Promising Places to Live, 1,200 Light-Years from Earth," with an illustration of one of these planets, looking just like Earth.[23] These are her thoughts:

> My reaction upon seeing this artist's rendering of this planet was to cringe. Then I felt nauseated. It was an immediate response, like an emotion of anger or joy, something we really don't have control over. It took a little while for me to realize why. This

planet, a place with water, clouds, a sun, warmth—an Earth lookalike literally and figuratively—represented the last ultimate place to move, to escape from all the pollution, the toxins, the destruction of our own planet. And this should make me happy, right? Like the people in the article, I should celebrate because maybe this planet supports life, and maybe it could support human life too.

And that's when I realized that my thought processes have changed drastically—they have become tainted, just like the water, air, and soil of those living in the middle of the industrial zones, in the communities where unconventional fossil fuel extraction is taking place. Four years of researching and documenting the lives of people and animals living in these communities has forced me to understand firsthand the consequences of our habitation and our endless thirst for fuel. Seeing this picture triggered an immediate cascade, like the fight-or-flight response. I see this new Earth, and instead of a great new place to live, I see it through the eyes of the fossil fuel industry—where are the sources of energy, where can we set the rigs, drill down, squeeze out as much fuel and as many dollars as possible?

It all occurred in a rush—this new potential Earth, clean and fresh, in an instant, became as our Earth, contaminated, toxic, screaming, as the last bits of fossil fuels are squeezed from her innards.

I ask if it has to be this way. If we could inhabit these new worlds, if we truly had a second chance, could we do it right the second time and inhabit the land without destroying it?

ACKNOWLEDGMENTS

We thank our editors, Alexis Rizzuto and Will Myers, and the staff of Beacon for helping to make this book a reality.

We would also like to thank James Muldoon, Kendra Smith, and David and Helen Slottje for advice on legal matters, Russell Galen for advice on literary contracts, Lou Allstadt for advice on the technical aspects of unconventional gas extraction, and Dr. Amy Seidl for advice on editors and agents. While exploring the subject of this book, we have met and come to know many wonderful people who have become our friends. Many of these people live in New York and Pennsylvania, but because unconventional fossil fuel extraction knows no bounds, we have also befriended people in California, Colorado, North Dakota, Texas, Arkansas, Louisiana, and Ohio. Although it would be impossible to list all of the people who have given us advice and helped over the last few years, we will mention a few: Dr. Jessica Ernst, Dr. Jan Zeserson, Dr. Hugh MacMillan, Dr. Leslie Walleigh, Dr. Larysa Dyrszka, Dr. Jannette Barth, Dr. Yuri Gorbi, Dr. John Stolz, Dr. Bryce Payne, Dr. Alisa Rich, Dr. Anthony Ingraffea, Dr. Robert Howarth, Dr. Motoko Mukai, Dr. Linda Nicholson, Dr. Gregory Weiland, Dr. Ron Bishop, Dr. Craig Slatin, Dr. William Podulka, Dr. Adam Law, Dr. Madelon Finkel, Dr. Julie Huntsman, Dr. Irene Weiser, Ron Gulla, Robert Donnan, Sandy Podulka, Sharon Wilson, William DuBose, Tara Meixsell, Lisa Bracken,

Rick Roles, Jake Hays, Hillary Acton, Elaine Hill, Nadia Steinzor, Krys Cail, Carol French, Claude Arnold, Carolyn Knapp, the UGDAB8 (Jane Penrose, Ann Furman, Ken Zeserson, Judy Abrams, Michael Dineen, and Jan Quarles), and our sons, Ben and Aaron Oswald.

We are most grateful to the families that participated in our research. They opened up their hearts and homes to us by agreeing to many hours of initial interviews and even more hours of visits and follow-up telephone calls and questions. Many of these people continue to give us updates, allowing us to glimpse what the long-term health impacts of living in the midst of unconventional fossil fuel operations looks like. Without these families and their animals, this book would not have been possible. Because this book does not include stories from all of the families we interviewed, and because each family's story could be a book in its own right, we hope that these families, and especially the children, will write their own stories, not only for themselves but also for future generations that may be faced with living in an industrial zone.

This book would not have been possible without the support, advice, and encouragement of Dr. Sandra Steingraber. Sandra is a constant source of inspiration who selflessly offered her time and insights from the beginning of this project all the way through to the end. We are most fortunate to have her as a neighbor, a colleague, and a friend.

NOTES

FOREWORD

1. L. Legere, "Sunday Times Review of DEP Drilling Records Reveals Water Damage, Murky Testing Methods," *Scranton (PA) Times-Tribune*, May 13, 2013, http://thetimes-tribune.com/news/sunday-times-review-of-dep-drilling -records-reveals-water-damage-murky-testing-methods-1.1491547.

2. A. Ingraffea, *Fluid Migration Mechanisms Due to Faulty Well Design and/or Construction: An Overview and Recent Experiences in the Pennsylvania Marcellus Play* (Ithaca, NY: Physicians, Scientists and Engineers for Healthy Energy, 2013), http://www.psehealthyenergy.org/data/PSE__Cement_Failure_Causes_and_ Rate_Analysis_Jan_2013_Ingraffea1.pdf.

3. Associated Press, "EPA Halted 'Fracking' Case After Gas Company Protested," January 16, 2013, http://www.usatoday.com/story/news/nation/2013/ 01/16/epa-gas-company-protested/1839857/; A. Rascoe, "EPA Ends Probe of Wyoming Water Pollution Linked to Fracking," Reuters, June 20, 2013, http:// www.reuters.com/article/2013/06/20/us-usa-epa-fracking-idUSBRE95 J1AN20130620.

4. J. Efstathiou Jr. and M. Drajem, "Drillers Silence Fracking Claims With Sealed Settlements," *Bloomberg News*, June 6, 2013, http://www.bloomberg .com/news/2013-06-06/drillers-silence-fracking-claims-with-sealed -settlements.html.

5. "Judge Defeats Challenge to 'Medical Gag Order' on Health Risks from Fracking," *RT*, October 31, 2013, http://rt.com/usa/medical-gag-rule-risks -fracking-053/.

INTRODUCTION

1. MAP-Tompkins, "The Marcellus Accountability Project for Tompkins County," 2010, www.tcgasmap.org/.

2. New York State, Environmental Conservation Law, "Environmental Conservation," section 23-0901, "Compulsory Integration and Unitization in Oil and Natural Gas Pools and Fields," accessed December 15, 2013, http://public.leginfo.state.ny.us/.

3. Centers for Disease Control, "Epidemiologic Aspects of the Current Outbreak of Kaposi's Sarcoma and Opportunistic Infections," *New England Journal of Medicine* 306 (1982): 248–52.

4. M. Bamberger and R.E. Oswald, "Impacts of Gas Drilling on Human and Animal Health," *New Solutions* 22 (2012): 51–77.

5. J.S. Campbell, "Flexible Driving Shaft," 1891, www.google.com/patents/US459152.

6. D.W. Lique, C.H. Cranston, and D.F. Morehouse, "Drilling Sideways: A Review of Horizontal Well Technology and Its Domestic Application," Energy Information Administration, Office of Oil and Gas, US Department of Energy, April 1993, www.eia.gov/pub/oil_gas/natural_gas/analysis_publications/drilling_sideways_well_technology/pdf/tr0565.pdf.

7. T.L. Watson, "Granites of the Southeastern Atlantic States," US Geological Survey, bulletin 426 (1910), http://pubs.usgs.gov/bul/0426/report.pdf.

8. Halliburton, "Hydraulic Fracturing 101," 2013, www.halliburton.com/public/projects/pubsdata/hydraulic_fracturing/fracturing_101.html.

9. New York State Department of Environmental Conservation, "Natural Gas Development Activities and High-Volume Hydraulic Fracturing," revised draft, Supplemental Generic Environmental Impact Statement, 2011, www.dec.ny.gov/docs/materials_minerals_pdf/rdsgeisch50911.pdf.

10. *Wikipedia*, s.v. "hydraulic fracturing," last modified December 19, 2013, http://en.wikipedia.org/wiki/Hydraulic_fracturing; Halliburton, "A Case Study: Sleeping Giant: The Story Behind the First Economically Successfuly Shale Play," 2012, www.halliburton.com/public/common/Case_Histories/H08944.pdf.

11. A. Messer, "Unconventional Natural Gas Reservoir Could Boost U.S. Supply," *Penn State News*, January 17, 2008, http://news.psu.edu/story/191364/2008/01/17/unconventional-natural-gas-reservoir-could-boost-us-supply.

12. US Geological Survey, "USGS Releases New Assessment of Gas Resources in the Marcellus Shale, Appalachian Basin," August 23, 2011, www.usgs.gov/newsroom/article.asp?ID=2893.

13. The estimate of six months is very crude and cannot be made with a great deal of confidence. This number was generated by using the percentage of gas extractable from counties in New York State, estimated by T. Engelder, "Marcellus," August 2009, www3.geosc.psu.edu/~jte2/references/link155.pdf,

and multiplying it by the total amount of gas estimated to be extractable from the Marcellus by US Geological Survey, "USGS Releases New Assessment."

14. L. W. Allstadt (former executive vice president of Mobil Oil Corporation responsible for exploration and production in the United States), personal communication, 2013.

15. A. E. Berman and L. F. Pittinger, "U.S. Shale Gas: Less Abundance, Higher Cost," *The Oil Drum*, August 5, 2011, www.theoildrum.com/node/8212.

16. A. Nikiforuk, *Saboteurs* (Toronto: Macfarlane Walter & Ross, 2011).

17. J. Gordon, "Canada Fracking Protests Turn Violent; 40 Arrested After Police Cars Set on Fire," *Huffington Post*, October 17, 2013, www.huffington post.com/2013/10/18/canada-fracking-protests_n_4118301.html.

18. C. L. Waldner, C. S. Ribble, E. D. Janzen, and J. R. Campbell, "Associations Between Oil- and Gas-Well Sites, Processing Facilities, Flaring, and Beef Cattle Reproduction and Calf Mortality in Western Canada," *Preventive Veterinary Medicine* 50 (July 19, 2001): 1–17; C. L. Waldner, "The Association Between Exposure to the Oil and Gas Industry and Beef Calf Mortality in Western Canada," *Archives of Occupational and Environmental Health* 63 (2008): 220–40; C. L. Waldner and E. G. Clark, "Association Between Exposure to Emissions From the Oil and Gas Industry and Pathology of the Immune, Nervous, and Respiratory Systems, and Skeletal and Cardiac Muscle in Beef Calves," *Archives of Occupational and Environmental Health* 64 (2009): 6–26; D. G. Bechtel, C. L. Waldner, and M. Wicktrom, "Associations Between In Utero Exposure to Airborne Emissions from Oil and Gas Production and Processing Facilities and Immune System Outcomes in Neonatal Beef Calves," *Archives of Occupational and Environmental Health* 64 (2009): 59–71; D. G. Bechtel, C. L. Waldner, and M. Wicktrom, "Associations Between Immune Function in Yearling Beef Cattle and Airborne Emissions of Sulfur Dioxide, Hydrogen Sulfide, and VOCs from Oil and Natural Gas Facilities," *Archives of Occupational and Environmental Health* 64 (2009): 73–86.

19. Ohio Oil and Gas Association, "Hydraulic Fracturing," accessed December 15, 2013, http://ooga.org/our-industry/hydraulic-fracturing/.

20. Associated Press, "Report: Drilling Damage in 161 Pa. Water Supplies," *Reporter News*, May 19, 2013, http://www.thereporteronline.com/article/RO/20130519/NEWS03/130519477.

21. "Fracking Experts Debate Economic, Environmental Impact," *Dundee (NY) Observer-Review*, 2013, www.observer-review.com/fracking-experts-debate-economic-environmental-impact-cms-3589.

22. C. Brufatto et al., "From Mud to Cement: Building Gas Wells," *Oilfield Review* (Schlumberger) (Autumn 2003): 62–76.

23. A. R. Ingraffea, "Fluid Migration Mechanisms Due to Faulty Well Design and/or Construction: An Overview and Recent Experiences in the Pennsylvania Marcellus Play," Physicians Scientists & Engineers for Healthy Energy,

January 2013, www.psehealthyenergy.org/data/PSE__Cement_Failure_Causes _and_Rate_Analysis_Jan_2013_Ingraffea1.pdf.

24. S. G. Osborn, A. Vengosh, N. R. Warner, and R. B. Jackson, "Methane Contamination of Drinking Water Accompanying Gas-Well Drilling and Hydraulic Fracturing," *Proceedings of the National Academy of Sciences USA* 108 (2011): 8172–76.

25. US Environmental Protection Agency (hereafter EPA), "Hydraulic Fracturing Background Information," last updated May 9, 2012, http://water .epa.gov/type/groundwater/uic/class2/hydraulicfracturing/wells_hydrowhat .cfm.

26. EPA, "Identification and Listing of Hazardous Waste," 40 CFR §261.4(b)(5) (2002).

27. EPA, "Draft Plan to Study the Potential Impacts of Hydraulic Fracturing on Drinking Water Resources," February 7, 2011, www2.epa.gov/hfstudy/ draft-plan-study-potential-impacts-hydraulic-fracturing-drinking-water -resources-february-7.

28. R. Beusse et al., "EPA Needs to Improve Air Emissions Data from the Oil and Natural Gas Production Sector," EPA, February 20, 2013, www.epa .gov/oig/reports/2013/20130220-13-P-0161.pdf.

29. This quote by Lisa Jackson was transcribed from the film *Gasland Part 2*, by Josh Fox (HBO, 2013).

30. C. R. Sunstein, *Laws of Fear: Beyond the Precautionary Principle* (Cambridge, UK: Cambridge University Press, 2005).

31. P. M. Rabinowitz, M. L. Scotch, and L. A. Conti, "Animals as Sentinels: Using Comparative Medicine to Move Beyond the Laboratory," *Institute of Laboratory Animal Resources Journal* 51, no. 3 (2010): 262–67.

32. Bamberger and Oswald, "Impacts of Gas Drilling on Human and Animal Health."

33. National Research Council, Commission on Life Sciences, Board on Environmental Studies and Toxicology, Committee on Animals as Monitors of Environmental Health Hazards, *Animals as Sentinels of Environmental Health Hazards* (Washington, DC: National Academy Press, 1991).

34. E. Hill, "Unconventional Natural Gas Development and Infant Health: Evidence from Pennsylvania," working paper 2012-12, Charles H. Dyson School of Applied Economics and Management, Cornell University, Ithaca, NY, July 2012, http://dyson.cornell.edu/research/researchpdf/wp/2012/ Cornell-Dyson-wp1212.pdf. See also L. M. McKenzie et al., "Birth Outcomes and Maternal Residential Proximity to Natural Gas Development in Rural Colorado," *Environmental Health Perspectives* (2014) http://dx.doi.org/10.1289/ ehp.1306722.

35. Centers for Disease Control and Prevention, NIOSH Program Portfolio,"Oil and Gas Extraction, Inputs: Occupational Safety and Health

Risks," last updated December 13, 2012, www.cdc.gov/niosh/programs/oilgas/risks.html.

ONE: FAMILIES AND THEIR PETS

1. Pediatric Environmental Health Specialty Units, PEHSU (2011), "PEHSU Information on Natural Gas Extraction and Hydraulic Fracturing for Health Professionals," August 2011, http://abcalliance.org/wp-content/uploads/2011/09/hydraulic_fracturing_and_children_2011_health_prof.pdf.

2. Stephanie Hallowich and Chris Hallowich, H/W v. Range Resources Corporation et al., Court of Common Pleas, Washington County, PA, Civil Division, Opinion and Order, March 20, 2013, available at http://earthjustice.org/sites/default/files/Hallowich-Opinion-Order.pdf.

3. Susan Phillips and Marie Cusick, "Drilling Companies Agree to Settle Fracking Contamination Case for $750,000," State Impact, March 21, 2013, http://stateimpact.npr.org/pennsylvania/2013/03/21/drilling-companies-agree-to-settle-fracking-contamination-case-for-750000.

4. Stephanie Hallowich and Chris Hallowich, H/W v. Range Resources Corporation et al., Court of Common Pleas, Washington County, PA, Civil Division, "Transcript of Inchambers Proceeding Before the Honorable Paul Pozonsky, Judge, on August 23, 2011," no. 2010-3954, http://ae3b703522cf9ac6c40a-32964bea949fe02d45161cf7095bfea9.r89.cf2.rackcdn.com/2013/211/626/pg-settlement-hearing-transcript.pdf.

5. K. Fisher and N. Warpinski, "Hydraulic Fracture Height Growth: Real Data," Society of Petroleum Engineers Production & Operations 27 (2012): 8–19.

6. R. E. Bishop, "Historical Analysis of Oil and Gas Well Plugging in New York: Is the Regulatory System Working?" New Solutions 23, no. 1 (2013): 103–16.

7. S. G. Osborn, A. Vengosh, N. R. Warner, and R. B. Jackson, "Methane Contamination of Drinking Water Accompanying Gas-Well Drilling and Hydraulic Fracturing," Proceedings of the National Academy of Sciences USA 108 (2011): 8172–76.

8. J. Hurdle, "Pennsylvania Report Left Out Data on Poisons in Water Near Gas Site," New York Times, November 2, 2012, www.nytimes.com/2012/11/03/us/pennsylvania-omitted-poison-data-in-water-report.html?_r=1&.

9. Environmental Protection Agency (EPA), "Drinking Water Contaminants," accessed December 15, 2013, http://water.epa.gov/drink/contaminants/index.cfm.

10. L. N. Vandenberg et al., "Hormones and Endocrine-Disrupting Chemicals: Low-Dose Effects and Nonmonotonic Dose Responses," Endocrine Reviews 33, no. 3 (2012): 378–455.

11. J. Treas, T. Tyagi, and K. P. Singh, "Chronic Exposure to Arsenic, Estrogen, and Their Combination Causes Increased Growth and Transformation

in Human Prostate Epithelial Cells Potentially by Hypermethylation-Mediated Silencing of MLH1," *Prostate* 73 (2013): 1660–72.

12. EPA, "Draft Plan to Study the Potential Impacts of Hydraulic Fracturing on Drinking Water Resources," February 7, 2011, www2.epa.gov/hfstudy/draft-plan-study-potential-impacts-hydraulic-fracturing-drinking-water-resources-february-7.

13. EPA, "Drinking Water Contaminants," accessed December 15, 2013, http://water.epa.gov/drink/contaminants/index.cfm.

14. EPA, "Regulating Public Water Systems and Contaminants Under the Safe Drinking Water Act," 2012, http://water.epa.gov/lawsregs/rulesregs/regulatingcontaminants/basicinformation.cfm.

15. G. Zhang et al., "Microbial Diversity in Ultra-High-Pressure Rocks and Fluids from the Chinese Continental Scientific Drilling Project in China," *Applied and Environmental Microbiology* 71 (2005): 3213–27.

TWO: SARAH AND JOSIE

1. Frac Technical Services International, "Material Safety Data Sheet, FRW-200," December 21, 2011, http://oilandgas.ohiodnr.gov/portals/oilgas/_MSDS/fractech/FRW-200.pdf.

2. A.R. Ingraffea, "Fluid Migration Mechanisms Due to Faulty Well Design and/or Construction: An Overview and Recent Experiences in the Pennsylvania Marcellus Play," Physicians Scientists and Engineers for Healthy Energy, February 18, 2013, www.psehealthyenergy.org/site/view/1057.

3. C. Brufatto et al., "From Mud to Cement: Building Gas Wells," *Oilfield Review* (Schlumberger) (autumn 2003): 62–76.

4. Pedro Ramirez Jr., *Reserve Pit Management: Risks to Migratory Birds* (Cheyenne, WY: US Fish and Wildlife Service, 2009), http://www.fws.gov/mountain-prairie/contaminants/documents/reservepits.pdf.

5. 25 PA code 488.435, 25 PA code 289.262.

6. Agency for Toxic Substances and Disease Registry, "Toxicological Profile for Hydrogen Sulfide," Toxic Substances Portal, July 2006, www.atsdr.cdc.gov/toxprofiles/tp.asp?id=389&tid=67.

7. Ibid.

8. Multi-Chem, Material Safety Data Sheet, MC B-8642, 2011.

9. For information on acrolein, see Science Lab, "Material Safety Data Sheet: Acrolein MSDS," last updated May 21, 2013, www.sciencelab.com/msds.php?msdsId=9922791. For glutaraldehyde, see Science Lab, "Material Safety Data Sheet: Glutaraldehyde Solution, 50% MSDS," last updated May 21, 2013, www.sciencelab.com/msds.php?msdsId=9924161.

10. Dystocia is a difficult or abnormal birth or labor.

11. OSHA, "Occupational Safety and Health Guidelines for Arsenic," www.osha.gov/SLTC/arsenic/index.html.

12. Pennsylvania Department of Environmental Protection, "Act 13 of 2012," accessed December 15, 2013, www.portal.state.pa.us/portal/server.pt/community/act_13/20789.

13. The New York State Department of Environmental Conservation provides a partial list of chemicals used in hydraulic fracturing fluid: "Natural Gas Development Activities and High-Volume Hydraulic Fracturing," chapter 5 in *Supplemental Generic Environmental Impact Statement*, revised draft (Albany: NYSDEC, 2011), www.dec.ny.gov/docs/materials_minerals_pdf/rdsgeisch509 11.pdf. Other information can be found at www.fracfocus.org.

14. Food & Water Watch, "Fracking: The New Global Water Crisis," March 2012, http://documents.foodandwaterwatch.org/doc/FrackingCrisisUS .pdf; SourceWatch "Fracking and Water Pollution," 2013, www.sourcewatch .org/index.php/Fracking_and_water_pollution.

15. Agency for Toxic Substances and Disease Registry, "Toxicological Profile for Arsenic," August 2007, www.atsdr.cdc.gov/toxprofiles/tp2.pdf; Agency for Toxic Substances and Disease Registry, "Health Consultation," October 29, 2013, www.atsdr.cdc.gov/HAC/pha/ChesapeakeATGASWellSite/Chesapeake ATGASWellSiteHC10282013_508.pdf.

16. EPA, "Chemicals in the Environment: Toluene (CAS No. 108-88-3)," August 1994, www.epa.gov/chemfact/f_toluene.txt.

17. M.A. D'Andrea and G.K. Reddy, "Health Effects of Benzene Exposure Among Children Following a Flaring Incident at the British Petroleum Refinery in Texas City," *Pediatric Hematology and Oncology* (October 2, 2013), DOI: 10.3109/08880018.2013.831511.

18. D. Campagna et al., "Color Vision and Occupational Toluene Exposure," *Neurotoxicol Teratol* 23 (2001): 473–80; E.H. Lee et al., "Acquired Dyschromatopsia Among Petrochemical Industry Workers Exposed to Benzene," *Neurotoxicology* 28 (2007): 356–63; MedlinePlus, "Benzene Poisoning," last updated February 16, 2012, www.nlm.nih.gov/medlineplus/ency/article/0027 20.htm.

19. L.W.D. Weber and J.T. Pierce, "Toxicology of Sensory Organs," in *Toxicology Principles for the Industrial Hygienist*, ed. W.E. Luttrell, W.W. Jederberg, and K.R. Still (Fairfax, VA: American Industrial Hygiene Association, 2008), 70–81.

20. Ibid.

21. Phenol and hippuric acid are imperfect markers because they can be found in the urine of individuals for reasons (e.g., eating some types of vegetables) other than direct exposure to benzene and toluene. However, Sarah and her family had multiple tests of their phenol and hippuric acid levels, and increased levels were correlated with time spent in their home. That is, the levels always dropped after they left their home for an extended time and increased when they spent time in their home.

22. "Range Resources Answers Question on Their Stinky Impoundment," video in two parts, YouTube, uploaded by "Cineplex Rex" on April 13, 2012, www.youtube.com/watch?v=QbWqR9KoVp4 and www.youtube.com/watch?v =GLpEMPzXWMY.

23. F. P. Perera et al., "Effect of Prenatal Exposure to Airborne Polycyclic Aromatic Hydrocarbons on Neurodevelopment in the First 3 Years of Life Among Inner-City Children," *Environmental Health Perspectives* 114 (2006): 1287–92; F. P. Perera et al., "Prenatal Airborne Polycyclic Aromatic Hydrocarbon Exposure and Child IQ at Age 5 Years," *Pediatrics* 124 (2009): e195–e202.

24. US Food and Drug Adminstration, "Protocol for Interpretation and Use of Sensory Testing and Analytical Chemistry Results for Re-opening Oil-Impacted Areas Closed to Seafood Harvesting Due to the Deepwater Horizon Oil Spill," 2010, www.fda.gov/food/ucm217601.htm.

25. EPA, "Draft Plan to Study the Potential Impacts of Hydraulic Fracturing on Drinking Water Resources," February 7, 2011, www2.epa.gov/hfstudy/ draft-plan-study-potential-impacts-hydraulic-fracturing-drinking-water -resources-february-7; T. Hayes, *Sampling and Analysis of Water Streams Associated with the Development of Marcellus Shale Gas* (Des Plaines, IL: Gas Technology Institute, 2009).

26. EPA, "Drinking Water Contaminants," accessed December 15, 2013, http://water.epa.gov/drink/contaminants, has this explanation: "Maximum Contaminant Level Goal (MCLG)—The level of a contaminant in drinking water below which there is no known or expected risk to health. MCLGs allow for a margin of safety and are non-enforceable public health goals. Maximum Contaminant Level (MCL)—The highest level of a contaminant that is allowed in drinking water. MCLs are set as close to MCLGs as feasible using the best available treatment technology and taking cost into consideration. MCLs are enforceable standards." On the same website, the EPA also defines secondary MCL standards: "National Secondary Drinking Water Regulations (NSDWRs or secondary standards) are non-enforceable guidelines regulating contaminants that may cause cosmetic effects (such as skin or tooth discoloration) or aesthetic effects (such as taste, odor, or color) in drinking water. EPA recommends secondary standards to water systems but does not require systems to comply. However, states may choose to adopt them as enforceable standards."

27. EPA, "Ethylene Glycol Monobutyl Ether (EGBE) (2-Butoxyethanol) (CASRN 111-76-2)," Integrated Risk Information System, March 31, 2010, www.epa.gov/iris/subst/0500.htm; US House of Representatives, Committee on Energy and Commerce, "Chemicals Used in Hydraulic Fracturing," April 2011, http://democrats.energycommerce.house.gov/sites/default/files/ documents/Hydraulic-Fracturing-Chemicals-2011-4-18.pdf.

28. National Toxicology Program, "Toxicology and Carcinogenesis Studies of 2-Butoxyethanol in F344/N Rats and B6C3F1 Mice," March 2000, http:// ntp.niehs.nih.gov/ntp/htdocs/lt_rpts/tr484.pdf.

THREE: SAMANTHA AND JESSE

1. L. Legere, "Hazards Posed by Natural Gas Drilling Not Always Underground," *Scranton (PA) Times-Tribune*, June 21, 2010, http://thetimes-tribune.com/news/hazards-posed-by-natural-gas-drilling-not-always-underground-1.857452.

2. Agency for Toxic Substances and Disease Registry, "Health Consultation," October 29, 2013, www.atsdr.cdc.gov/HAC/pha/ChesapeakeATGAS WellSite/ChesapeakeATGASWellSiteHC10282013_508.pdf.

3. S. G. Osborn, A. Vengosh, N. R. Warner, and R. B. Jackson, "Methane Contamination of Drinking Water Accompanying Gas-Well Drilling and Hydraulic Fracturing," *Proceedings of the National Academy of Sciences USA* 108 (2011): 8172–76.

4. K. K. Eltschlager, J. W. Hawkins, W. C. Ehler, and F. Baldassare, "Technical Measures for the Investigation and Mitigation of Fugitive Methane Hazards in Areas of Coal Mining," US Department of the Interior, Office of Surface Mining Reclamation and Enforcement, Pittsburgh, September 2001.

5. Centers for Disease Control and Prevention, NIOSH Program Portfolio, "Oil and Gas Extraction. Inputs: Occupational Safety and Health Risks," last updated December 13, 2012, www.cdc.gov/niosh/programs/oilgas/risks.html.

6. A. R. Ingraffea, "Insights on Unconventional Natural Gas Development from Shale: An Interview with Anthony R. Ingraffea by Adam Law," *New Solutions* 23, no. 1 (2013): 203 8.

7. StateImpact Pennsylvania, "Well: Morse 5H," Shale Play, Natural Gas Drilling in Pennsylvania, accessed December 15, 2013, http://stateimpact.npr.org/pennsylvania/drilling/wells/015-20932/; L. Kasianowitz, Information Specialist and South-central Community Relations Coordinator, Pennsylvania Department of Environmental Protection, personal communication, September 30, 2013.

8. Gas Safety Incorporated, "Report to Damascus Citizens for Sustainability and Mr. Don Williams on 25 July 2012 Field Inspection and Methane Sampling Survey of Parts of Leroy, Granville and Franklin Townships Bradford County, Pennsylvania," accessed December 15, 2013, www.damascuscitizens forsustainability.org/wp-content/uploads/2012/08/Leroy2-072512-report-FINAL.pdf.

FOUR: ANN AND ANDREW

1. G. Albrecht et al., "Solastalgia: The Distress Caused by Environmental Change," *Australas Psychiatry* 15 suppl. 1 (2007): S95–S98.

2. H. E. Bergna, "Petroleum Refinery Processes Using Catalyst of Aluminosilicate Sols and Powders," 1981, Patent US 4257874 A, www.google.com/patents/US4257874.

3. J.L. Hewitt, "The Levant Investigation: Using Radiocarbon Dating to Determine the Source of Methane Gas Migration," 1984, info.ngwa.org/gwol/pdf/870143442.PDF.

FIVE: FRACKING, FARMING, AND OUR FOOD SUPPLY

1. W. Hauter, *Foodopoly: The Battle over the Future of Food and Farming in America* (New York: New Press, 2012); D. Kirby, *Animal Factory: The Looming Threat of Industrial Pig, Dairy, and Poultry Farms to Humans and the Environment* (New York: St. Martin's Griffin, 2010).

2. General Assembly of Pennsylvania, House Bill 1950, Session of 2011, Report of the Committee of Conference, www.ctbpls.com/www/PA/11R/PDF/PA11RHB01950CC1.pdf.

3. State Review of Oil and Natural Gas Envronmental Regulations, Inc. (STRONGER), *Follow-Up State Review*, September 2013, http://strongerinc.org/sites/all/themes/stronger02/downloads/Final%20Report%20of%20Pennsylvania%20State%20Review%20Approved%20for%20Publication.pdf.

4. New York State Department of Environmental Conservation, "Natural Gas Development Activities and High-Volume Hydraulic Fracturing," revised draft, Supplemental Generic Environmental Impact Statement, 2011, www.dec.ny.gov/docs/materials_minerals_pdf/rdsgeisch50911.pdf.

5. New York State, Environmental Conservation Law, section 23-0901, "Compulsory Integration and Unitization in Oil and Natural Gas Pools and Fields," 2005, http://law.onecle.com/new-york/environmental-conservation/ENV023-0901_23-0901.html.

6. In 2008, Thomas S. West was the founder and managing partner of the West Firm.

7. New York State Senate, "Compulsory Integration Legislation," 2005, http://catskillcitizens.org/learnmore/CIO5.pdf.

8. New York State Department of Environmental Conservation, "Oil and Gas," webpage, accessed December 15, 2013, www.dec.ny.gov/energy/205.html. DEC's Division of Mineral Resources administers regulations and a permitting program to mitigate to the greatest extent possible any potential environmental impact of drilling and well operation. See "Regulated Well Types" on the right of the aforementioned web page, to get more details on which wells require permits, "Well Permitting Process" for instructions on how to apply for a permit, and "Forms" for all the required paperwork. In addition, the division protects the correlative rights of mineral owners and ensures that oil and gas reserves are developed such that a greater ultimate recovery can be achieved. This is accomplished through well spacing and compulsory integration.

9. State of Pennsylvania, "Oil and Gas Conservation Law, Act 1961-359, Laws of Pennsylvania, No. 1961-359, Unofficial Version," 1961, http://files.dep.state.pa.us/OilGas/BOGM/BOGMPortalFiles/LawsRegsGuidelines/Act359uc.pdf.

10. The "Onondaga horizon" is the top of the geological layer made of hard limestones and dolostones called the "Onondaga formation." For the most part, it lies below the Marcellus shale and outcrops to the surface in a line roughly running from Detroit, above Lake Erie, through Buffalo and Syracuse to Albany, New York.

11. Pennsylvania General Assembly, 2013 Act 66, "Oil and Gas Lease Act: Payment Information to Interest Owners for Accumulation of Proceeds from Production, Apportionment and Conflicts," July 9, 2013, www.legis.state.pa.us/cfdocs/legis/li/uconsCheck.cfm?yr=2013&sessInd=0&act=66.

12. The Pennsylvania Code, "Chapter 137b. Preferential Assessment of Farmland and Forest Land Under the Clean and Green Act," accessed December 15, 2013, www.pacode.com/secure/data/007/chapter137b/chap137btoc.html.

13. Argonne National Laboratory, Environmental Sciences Division, "Drilling Waste Management Information System, Fact Sheet: Land Application," accessed December 15, 2013, http://web.ead.anl.gov/dwm/techdesc/land/index.cfm; M.B. Adams, "Land Application of Hydrofracturing Fluids Damages a Deciduous Forest Stand in West Virginia," *Journal of Environmental Quality* 40 (2011): 1340–44.

14. EPA, "Radioactive Wastes from Oil and Gas Drilling," last updated August 14, 2012, www.epa.gov/radtown/drilling-waste.html.

15. Radio New Zealand News, "Fonterra to Stop Taking Milk from Farms with Oil and Gas Waste," June 19, 2013, www.radionz.co.nz/news/rural/138025/fonterra-to-stop-taking-milk-from-farms-with-oil-and-gas-waste.

16. R. Udall, "The Shale Phenomenon: Fabulous Miracle with a Fatal Flaw," *Christian Science Monitor*, February 22, 2013, www.csmonitor.com/Environment/Energy-Voices/2013/0222/The-shale-phenomenon-fabulous-miracle-with-a-fatal-flaw.

17. Lundberg Family Farms. "Understanding Arsenic in Food," 2013, www.lundberg.com/info/Arsenic.aspx.

18. D. Hvinden, "So Why Are All These Gas Flares Burning in the Oil Fields?" *North Dakota Department of Mineral Resources Newsletter* 36 (2009): 5–6.

19. Earthworks Action, "Deborah Rogers," *Earthworks*, accessed December 15, 2013, www.earthworksaction.org/voices/detail/deborah_rogers.

20. M. Moss, *Salt Sugar Fat: How the Food Giants Hooked Us* (New York: Random House, 2013).

21. Louisiana Department of Environmental Quality, Case AI No. 164544, 2010, http://edms.deq.louisiana.gov/app/doc/querydef.aspx.

22. M. Bamberger and R. E. Oswald, "Impacts of Gas Drilling on Human and Animal Health," *New Solutions* 22 (2012): 51–77.

23. Ibid.

24. L. N. Vandenberg et al., "Hormones and Endocrine-Disrupting Chemicals: Low-Dose Effects and Nonmonotonic Dose Responses," *Endocrine Reviews* 33, no. 3 (2012): 378–455.

25. Agency for Toxic Substances and Disease Registry, "Toxic Substances Portal: Strontium," April 2004, www.atsdr.cdc.gov/phs/phs.asp?id=654&tid=120.

26. EPA, "Radium," last updated March 6, 2012, www.epa.gov/radiation/radionuclides/radium.html.

27. Bamberger and Oswald, "Impacts of Gas Drilling."

28. US Department of Agriculture, "National Organic Program," last modified January 31, 2011, www.ams.usda.gov/AMSv1.0/ams.fetchTemplateData.do?template=TemplateF&leftNav=NationalOrganicProgram&page=NOPResourceCenterRegulations&description=NOP Regulations.

29. For PAH testing, see US Food and Drug Administration, "Protocol for Interpretation and Use of Sensory Testing and Analytical Chemistry Results for Re-opening Oil-Impacted Areas Closed to Seafood Harvesting Due to the Deepwater Horizon Oil Spill," June 2010, www.fda.gov/food/ucm217601.htm. For DOSS testing, see R.A. Flurer et al., "Determination of Dioctylsulfosuccinate in Select Seafoods Using a QuEChERS Extraction with Liquid Chromatography-Triple Quadrupole Mass Spectrometry," *US Food and Drug Administration Laboratory Information Bulletin*, October 27, 2010, www.fda.gov/downloads/ScienceResearch/FieldScience/UCM231510.pdf.

30. Ibid.

31. A. Luch, *The Carcinogenic Effects of Polycyclic Aromatic Hydrocarbons* (London: Imperial College Press, 2005).

32. F. P. Perera et al., "Effect of Prenatal Exposure to Airborne Polycyclic Aromatic Hydrocarbons on Neurodevelopment in the First 3 Years of Life Among Inner-City Children," *Environmental Health Perspectives* 114 (2006): 1287–92; F. P. Perera et al., "Prenatal Airborne Polycyclic Aromatic Hydrocarbon Exposure and Child IQ at Age 5 Years," *Pediatrics* 124 (2009): e195–e202; S. C. Edwards et al., "Prenatal Exposure to Airborne Polycyclic Aromatic Hydrocarbons and Children's Intelligence at 5 Years of Age in a Prospective Cohort Study in Poland," *Environmental Health Perspectives* 118 (2010): 1326–31; F.P. Perera, W. Jedrychowski, V. Rauh, and R.M Whyatt, "Molecular Epidemiologic Research on the Effects of Environmental Pollutants on the Fetus," *Environmental Health Perspectives* 107, suppl. 3 (1999): 451–60; F. P. Perera et al., "Prenatal Polycyclic Aromatic Hydrocarbon (PAH) Exposure and Child Behavior at Age 6–7 Years," *Environmental Health Perspectives* 120 (2012): 921–26.

33. EPA, "Draft Plan to Study the Potential Impacts of Hydraulic Fracturing on Drinking Water Resources," February 7, 2011, www2.epa.gov/hfstudy/draft-plan-study-potential-impacts-hydraulic-fracturing-drinking-water-resources-february-7; Hayes, *Sampling and Analysis of Water Streams Associated with the Development of Marcellus Shale Gas*; US House of Representatives, Committee on Energy and Commerce, "Chemicals Used in Hydraulic Fractur-

ing," April 2011, http://democrats.energycommerce.house.gov/sites/default/files/documents/Hydraulic-Fracturing-Chemicals-2011-4-18.pdf; T. Colborn, C. Kwiatkowski, K. Schultz, and M. Bachran, "Natural Gas Operations from a Public Health Perspective," *International Journal of Human and Ecological Risk Assessment* 17 (2011): 1039–56; The Endocrine Disruption Exchange (TEDX), "Health Effects Spreadsheet and Summary," http://endocrinedisruption.org/chemicals-in-natural-gas-operations/chemicals-and-health .

34. EPA, "Draft Plan"; Hayes, *Sampling and Analysis of Water Streams Associated with the Development of Marcellus Shale Gas.*

35. Agency for Toxic Substances and Disease Registry, "Toxicological Profile for Radium," 2011, www.atsdr.cdc.gov/toxprofiles/tp.asp?id=791&tid=154; S. Bonotto, "Radium Uptake by Marine Plants," in *The Environmental Behaviour of Radium*, ed. IAEA (Vienna: International Atomic Energy Agency, 1990), 451–66; L. D. Hamilton, A. F. Meinhold, and J. Nagy, "Health Risk Assessment for Radium Discharged in Produced Waters," *Produced Water, Environmental Science Research* 46 (1992): 303–14; J. Justyn and B. Havlik, "Radium Uptake by Freshwater Fish," in *The Environmental Behaviour of Radium*, 529–43; S. L. Simon and S. A. Ibrahim, "Biological Uptake of Radium by Terrestrial Plants," in *The Environmental Behaviour of Radium*, 545–99; A. P. Watson, E. L. Etnier, and L. M. McDowell-Boyer, "Radium-226 in Drinking Water and Terrestrial Food Chains: Transfer Parameters and Normal Exposure and Dose," *Nuclear Safety* 25 (1984): 815–29; A. O. Bettencourt, M. M. G. R. Teixeira, M. D. T. Elias, and M. C. Faisca, "Soil to Plant Transfer of Radium-226," *Journal of Environmental Radioactivity* 6 (1988): 49–60.

36. N. R. Warner, C. A. Christie, R. B. Jackson, and A. Vengosh, "Impacts of Shale Gas Wastewater Disposal on Water Quality in Western Pennsylvania," *Environonmental Science and Technology* 47 (2013): 11849–57.

37. Ibid.

38. Technologicaly Enhanced Naturally Occurring Radioactive Material (TENORM), "U.S. Guidance," last updated December 13, 2013, www.tenorm.com/regs2.htm.

39. W. D. Hueston, "BSE and Variant CJD: Emerging Science, Public Pressure and the Vagaries of Policy-Making," *Preventive Veterinary Medicine* 109 (2013): 179–84.

40. G. Burke, "Colorado's Fracking Woes Show Fight Brewing in Oklahoma, Texas and Other Drought-Ridden Areas," *Huffington Post*, June 16, 2013, www.huffingtonpost.com/2013/06/16/colorado-fracking_n_3450170.html.

41. M. Freyman and R. Salmon, "Hydraulic Fracturing & Water Stress: Growing Competitive Pressures for Water," 2013, www.ceres.org/resources/reports/hydraulic-fracturing-water-stress-growing-competitive-pressures-for-water/view.

SIX: MARY AND CHARLIE

1. PA Canyon, http://pacanyon.com/.

2. Leases typically expire in five years, but automatically renew for another five, unless the owner has a special clause inserted.

3. Justin Fleming, "Cattle from Tioga County Farm Quarantined After Coming in Contact with Natural Gas Drilling Wastewater," Pennsylvania Department of Environmental Protection, Newsroom page, July 1, 2010, www.portal.state.pa.us/portal/server.pt/community/newsroom/14287?id=12588& typeid=1.

4. Food Animal Residue Avoidance Databank (FARAD), home page, accessed December 15, 2013, www.farad.org/.

5. Fleming, "Cattle from Tioga County Farm."

6. US Department of Energy Office of Fossil Energy and National Energy Technology Laboratory, *Modern Shale Gas Development in the United States: A Primer* (Oklahoma City: US Department of Energy and National Energy Technology Laboratory, April 2009), www.netl.doe.gov/technologies/oil-gas/ publications/EPreports/Shale_Gas_Primer_2009.pdf.

7. Pennsylvania Department of Environmental Protection, "Laws, Regulations and Guidelines," 2013, www.portal.state.pa.us/portal/server.pt/commu nity/laws,_regulations___guidelines/20306.

8. Fleming, "Cattle from Tioga County Farm."

9. Agency for Toxic Substances and Disease Registry, "Toxic Substances Portal: Strontium," April 2004, www.atsdr.cdc.gov/phs/phs.asp?id=654&tid =120.

10. H.F. Mayland, G.E. Shewmaker, and R.C. Bull, "Soil Ingestion by Cattle Grazing Crested Wheatgrass," *Journal of Range Management* 30 (1977): 264–65; A.L. Pope et al., "The Effect of Sulphur on 75Se Absorption and Retention in Sheep," *Journal of Nutrition* 109 (1979): 1448–55; J.W. Spears, "Trace Mineral Bioavailability in Ruminants," *Journal of Nutrition* 133 (2003): 1506S–1509S; H.F. Hintz and D.E. Hogue, "Effect of Selenium, Sulfur and Sulfur Amino Acids on Nutritional Muscular Dystrophy in the Lamb," *Journal of Nutrition* 82 (1964): 495–98; G.G. Fries, G.S. Marrow, and P.A. Snow, "Soil Ingestion by Dairy Cattle," *Journal of Dairy Science* 65 (1982): 611–18; J. Ivancic Jr. and W.P. Weiss, "Effect of Dietary Sulfur and Selenium Concentrations on Selenium Balance of Lactating Holstein Cows," *Journal of Dairy Science* 84 (2001): 225–32.

11. L.J. Hutchinson, R.W. Scholz, and T.R. Drake, "Nutritional Myodegeneration in a Group of Chianina Heifers," *Journal of the American Veterinary Medical Association* 181 (1982): 581–84; J.P. Orr and B.R. Blakley, "Investigation of the Selenium Status of Aborted Calves with Cardiac Failure and Mycardial Necrosis," *Journal of Veterinary Diagnostic Investigation* 9 (1997): 172–79.

12. Commonwealth of Pennsylvania Department of Agriculture, Right-to-

Know Law Request No. 111012, Veterinary Report Dated June 24, 2010: Memo to Dr. Anthony Labarbera from Dr. Amy Nestlerodt. Subject: Frac Water Holding Pond Still on Beef Farm in Tioga County.

13. Agency for Toxic Substances and Disease Registry, "Toxic Substances Portal: Strontium."

14. T. Colborn, C. Kwiatkowski, K. Schultz, and M. Bachran, "Natural Gas Operations from a Public Health Perspective," *International Journal of Human and Ecological Risk Assessment* 17 (2011): 1039–56.

15. Ibid.

16. M. B. Adams, "Land Application of Hydrofracturing Fluids Damages a Deciduous Forest Stand in West Virginia," *Journal of Environmental Quality* 40 (2011): 1340–44.

SEVEN: SHARON AND WADE

1. US Department of Agriculture, "USDA Census of Agriculture," accessed December 15, 2013, www.agcensus.usda.gov/index.php.

2. Cornell Cooperative Extension, "Calf Diseases and Prevention," January 14, 2011, www.extension.org/pages/15695/calf-diseases-and-prevention; S. Godden, "Calf Health Management," http://www.prpc.cog.tx.us/Programs/RegionalServices/Calf-Ranch-Industry/PRPC_CalfRanch/bioref/calf%20health%20managment%20ogodden.pdf.

3. H. S. Thomas, "BVD Is the Most Costly Viral Disease in Cattle," *Cattle Today*, October 2006, www.cattletoday.com/archive/2006/October/CT642.shtml; H. Bielefeldt-Ohmann, "An Ocular-Cerebellar Syndrome Caused by Congenital Viral Diarrhea Virus Infection," *Acta Veterinaria Scandinavica* 25 (1984): 36–49.

4. T. Colborn, C. Kwiatkowski, K. Schultz, and M. Bachran, "Natural Gas Operations from a Public Health Perspective," *International Journal of Human and Ecological Risk Assessment* 17 (2011): 1039–56; The Endocrine Disruption Exchange (TEDX), "Health Effects Spreadsheet and Summary," http://endocrinedisruption.org/chemicals-in-natural-gas-operations/chemicals-and-health; IPIECA, "Drilling Fluids and Health Risk Management," September 2009, www.ipieca.org/publication/drilling-fluids-and-health-risk-management; C. D. Kassotis, D. E. Tillitt, J. Wade Davis, A. M. Hormann, and S. C. Nagel, "Estrogen and Androgen Receptor Activities of Hydraulic Fracturing Chemicals and Surface and Ground Water in a Drilling-Dense Region," *Endocrinology* (2014): doi:10.1210/en.2013-1697.

EIGHT: ENVIRONMENTAL JUSTICE

1. EPA, "Environmental Justice," last updated November 19, 2013, http://www.epa.gov/environmentaljustice/.

2. J. M. Barth, "The Economic Impact of Shale Gas Development on State

and Local Economies: Benefits, Costs, and Uncertainties," *New Solutions* 23 (2013): 85–101.

3. US Supreme Court, Reynolds v. Sims, 377 US 533 (1964), http://supreme.justia.com/cases/federal/us/377/533/case.html.

4. New York State, Environmental Conservation Law, "Environmental Conservation," section 23-0303, "Administration of Article," accessed December 15, 2013, http://law.oncle.com/new-york/environmental-conservation/ENV023-0303_23-0303.html.

5. State of New York Supreme Court Appellate Division Third Judicial Department, In the Matter of Norse Energy Corporation USA v. Town of Dryden et al., Dryden Resources Awareness Coalition, decided and entered May 2, 2013, http://earthjustice.org/sites/default/files/Dryden-Decision.pdf.

6. "Norse Energy Corp ASA Announces Liquidation of United States Units-DJ," Reuters, October 11, 2013, http://in.reuters.com/finance/stocks/NEC.OL/key-developments/article/2846203.

7. Pennsylvania Department of Environmental Protection, "Act 13 of 2012," accessed December 15, 2013, www.portal.state.pa.us/portal/server.pt/community/act_13/20789.

8. President Judge Pellegrini (2012) Robinson Township, Washington County, Pennsylvania, Brian Coppola, Individually and in His Official Capacity as Supervisor of Robinson Township, Township of Nockamixon, Bucks County, Pennsylvania, Township of South Fayette, Allegheny County, Pennsylvania, Peters Township, Washington County, Pennsylvania, David M. Ball, Individually and in His Official Capacity as Councilman of Peters Township, Township of Cecil, Washington County, Pennsylvania, Mount Pleasant Township, Washington County, Pennsylvania, Borough of Yardley, Bucks County, Pennsylvania, Delaware Riverkeeper Network, Maya Van Rossum, the Delaware Riverkeeper, Mehernosh Khan, MD, Petitioners v. Pennsylvania Public Utility Commission, Robert F. Powelson, in His Official Capacity as Chairman of the Public Utility Commission, Office of the Attorney General of Pennsylvania, Linda L. Kelly, in Her Official Capacity as Attorney General of the Commonwealth of Pennsylvania, Pennsylvania Department of Environmental Protection and Michael L. Krancer, in His Official Capacity as Secretary of the Department of Environmental Protection, Respondents, filed July 26, 2012, http://s3.documentcloud.org/documents/404267/stateimpact-pennsylvania-act-13-ruling.pdf.

9. M. Kakareka, "Lawsuit Dropped Against Town of Sanford," *Time Warner Cable News, Central New York*, April 18, 2013, http://centralny.ynn.com/content/top_stories/657645/lawsuit-dropped-against-town-of-sanford/.

10. G. Ball, "New York State Senator Greg Ball," accessed December 15, 2013, www.nysenate.gov/senator/greg-ball.

11. White House, "Obama Administration Announces Comprehensive Strategy for Energy Security," news release, March 31, 2010, www.whitehouse

.gov/the-press-office/obama-administration-announces-comprehensive
-strategy-energy-security.

NINE: CLAIRE AND JASON

1. EPA, "Investigation of Ground-Water Contamination near Pavillion, Wyoming," 2011, www.epa.gov/region8/superfund/wy/pavillion/Nov30–2011_WorkgroupPresentation.pdf.

2. Fisher Scientific, "Material Safety Data Sheet: Bentonite," http://www.fishersci.in/msds/Bentonitepowder.pdf.

3. Agency for Toxic Substances and Disease Registry, "Toxicological Profile for Benzene," August 2007, www.atsdr.cdc.gov/toxprofiles/tp3-p.pdf.

4. Platelet Research Laboratory, "Platelet Function," last updated July 28, 2013, www.platelet-research.org/1/function_hemo.htm.

5. American Red Cross, "Guide for Shelter Managers," February 1988, www.region4a-mrc.org/documents/2009march/AMERICAN RED CROSS GUIDE FOR SHELTER MANAGERS.htm.

6. Many intensively drilled communities are in need of water donations: Water for Woodlands, "Water Needed," accessed December 15, 2013, https://sites.google.com/site/waterforwoodlands/home; Western Resource Advocates, "Fracking Our Future: Where's the Water?" accessed December 15, 2013, www.westernresourceadvocates.org/frackwater/; Citizens for Clean Water (clscraigstevens@earthlink.net); Berks Gas Truth, home page, accessed December 15, 2013, www.gastruth.org.

EPILOGUE

1. Louisiana Department of Environmental Quality, Case AI No. 164544, 2010, http://edms.deq.louisiana.gov/app/doc/querydef.aspx.

2. J. Karha and E. J. Topol, "The Sad Story of Vioxx, and What We Should Learn from It," *Cleveland Clinic Journal of Medicine* 71 (2004): 933–39.

3. *Toxic Ignorance* (Washington, DC: Environmental Defense Fund, 1997), www.edf.org.

4. Climate Central, *Global Weirdness: Severe Storms, Deadly Heat Waves, Relentless Drought, Rising Seas, and the Weather of the Future* (New York: Pantheon Books, 2013).

5. D. T. Shindell et al., "Improved Attribution of Climate Forcing to Emissions," *Science* 326 (2009): 716–18.

6. "Energy: Deep Sigh of Relief," *Economist*, March 16, 2013, www.economist.com/news/special-report/21573279-shale-gas-and-oil-bonanza-transforming-americas-energy-outlook-and-boosting-its%60o.

7. A. Nikiforuk, *The Energy of Slaves: Oil and the New Servitude* (Vancouver: Greystone Books, 2012).

8. International Monetary Fund, "Energy Subsidy Reform: Lessons and Implications," January 28, 2013, www.imf.org/external/np/pp/eng/2013/012813 .pdf.

9. Management Information Services, "60 Years of Energy Incentives: Analysis of Federal Expenditures for Energy Development," October 2011, www.nei.org/corporatesite/media/filefolder/60_Years_of_Energy_Incentives_ -_Analysis_of_Federal_Expenditures_for_Energy_Development_-_1950-2010 .pdf.

10. State of New York Supreme Court Appellate Division Third Judicial Department, In the Matter of Norse Energy Corporation USA v. Town of Dryden et al., Dryden Resources Awareness Coalition, decided and entered May 2, 2013, http://earthjustice.org/sites/default/files/Dryden-Decision.pdf.

11. N. Pfund and B. Healey, *What Would Jefferson Do? The Historical Role of Federal Subsidies in Shaping America's Energy Future* (San Francisco: DBL Investors, September 2011), www.dblinvestors.com/wp-content/uploads/2012/09/ What-Would-Jefferson-Do-2.4.pdf?597435&24e536.

12. M. Z. Jacobson et al., "Examining the Feasibility of Converting New York State's All-Purpose Energy Infrastructure to One Using Wind, Water, and Sunlight," *Energy Policy* 57 (2013): 585–601.

13. Federal Ministry for the Environment, Nature Conservation and Nuclear Safety, *Renewable Energy Sources in Figures: National and International Development* (Berlin: Federal Ministry for the Environment, Nature Conservation and Nuclear Safety, July 2013), http://www.bmu.de/fileadmin/Daten_BMU/ Pools/Broschueren/ee_in_zahlen_en_bf.pdf.

14. Ecovillage at Ithaca, "Renewable Energy," 2013, http://ecovillageithaca .org/evi/index.php/about/renewable-energy.

15. Solar Washington, "Bainbridge Island City Hall Community Solar Project," 2013, http://solarwa.org/tour/bainbridge-island/bainbridge-island -city-hall-community-solar-project.

16. Solarize New York, "Community Empowerment Through Collective Bargaining," 2013, www.solarizenewyork.org/.

17. US Department of Energy, "New York Incentives/Policies for Renewables & Efficiency: Net Metering," 2012, www.dsireusa.org/incentives/ incentive.cfm?Incentive_Code=NY05R.

18. E. Bruns, D. Ohlhorst, B. Wenzel, and J. Köppel, *Renewable Energies in Germany's Electricity Market: A Biography of the Innovation Process* (New York: Springer, 2011).

19. Passive House Institute, "The Independent Institute for Outstanding Energy Efficiency in Buildings," 2012, http://passiv.de/en/.

20. A. Kerr, "Plug-In Vehicles: Ready for Prime Time?" *Home Power* 151 (2012): 102–8.

APPENDIX

1. B.B. Van Diver, *Roadside Geology of New York* (Missoula, MT: Mountain Press Publishing, 1985).

2. A. Nikiforuk, *Tar Sands: Dirty Oil and the Future of a Continent* (Vancouver: Greystone Books, 2010).

3. *Wikipedia*, s.v. "Marcellus Formation," last modified December 26, 2013, http://en.wikipedia.org/wiki/Marcellus_Formation.

4. New York State Department of Environmental Conservation, "Geology," September 30, 2009, www.dec.ny.gov/docs/materials_minerals_pdf/ogds geischap4.pdf.

5. *Wikipedia*, s.v. "Utica Shale," last modified October 23, 2013, http://en.wikipedia.org/wiki/Utica_Shale.

6. Marcellus Center for Outreach and Research (MCOR), "Wet-Dry Gas," 2009, www.marcellus.psu.edu/images/Wet-Dry_Line_with_Depth.gif.

7. "Energy: Deep Sigh of Relief," *Economist*, March 16, 2013, www.economist.com/news/special-report/21573279-shale-gas-and-oil-bonanza-transforming-americas-energy-outlook-and-boosting-its%60o.

8. D. Hvinden, "So Why Are All These Gas Flares Burning in the Oil Fields?" *North Dakota Department of Mineral Resources Newsletter* 36 (2009): 5–6.

9. C. Krauss, "Oil Companies Are Sued for Waste of Natural Gas," *New York Times*, October 17, 2013, www.nytimes.com/2013/10/18/business/energy-environment/oil-companies-are-sued-over-natural-gas-flaring-in-north-dakota.html.

10. Chesapeake Energy, "Hydraulic Fracturing Fact Sheet," May 2012, http://www.chk.com/media/educational-library/fact-sheets/corporate/hydraulic_fracturing_fact_sheet.pdf.

11. Quoted in J. Goodell, "Rolling Stone Responds to Chesapeake Energy on 'The Fracking Bubble,'" *Rolling Stone*, March 6, 2012, www.rollingstone.com/politics/blogs/national-affairs/rolling-stone-responds-to-chesapeake-energy-on-the-fracking-bubble-20120306.

12. K. Fisher and N. Warpinski, "Hydraulic Fracture Height Growth: Real Data," *Society of Petroleum Engineers Production & Operations* 27 (2012): 8–19.

13. R.E. Bishop, "Historical Analysis of Oil and Gas Well Plugging in New York: Is the Regulatory System Working?" *New Solutions* 23, no. 1 (2013): 103–16.

14. S. Detrow, "Perilous Pathways: How Drilling Near an Abandoned Well Produced a Methane Geyser," *State Impact*, October 9, 2012, http://stateimpact.npr.org/pennsylvania/2012/10/09/perilous-pathways-how-drilling-near-an-abandoned-well-produced-a-methane-geyser/.

15. N.R. Warner et al., "Geochemical Evidence for Possible Natural Migration of Marcellus Formation Brine to Shallow Aquifers in Pennsylvania," *Proceedings of the National Academy of Sciences USA* 109 (2013): 11961–66.

16. C. D. Volz, "Natural Gas Drilling, Public Health and Environmental Impacts," Senate Committee on Environment and Public Works and Its Subcommittee on Water and Wildlife, Joint Hearing, 2011.

17. N. R. Warner, C. A. Christie, R. B. Jackson, and A. Vengosh, "Impacts of Shale Gas Wastewater Disposal on Water Quality in Western Pennsylvania," *Environonmental Science and Technology* 47 (2013): 11849–57.

18. K. M. Keranen, H. M. Savage, G. A. Abers, and E. S. Cochran, "Potentially Induced Earthquakes in Oklahoma, USA: Links Between Wastewater Injection and the 2011 Mw 5.7 Earthquake Sequence," *Geology* 41 (2013): 699–702.

19. W. L. Ellsworth et al., "Are Seismicity Rate Changes in the Midcontinent Natural or Manmade?" abstract of presentation given at Seismological Society of America, San Diego, April 18, 2012, http://tinyurl.com/7on2klp/.

20. Tight Oil Reservoirs California 2012, "Monterey & Surrounding Sediments," www.tight-oil-monterey-california-2012.com/.

21. D. Rogers, "Shale and Wall Street: Was the Decline in Natural Gas Prices Orchestrated?" February 2013, http://shalebubble.org/wp-content/uploads/2013/02/SWS-report-FINAL.pdf.

22. Barth, "The Economic Impact of Shale Gas Development."

23. D. Overbye, "Two Promising Places to Live, 1,200 Light-Years from Earth," *New York Times*, April 18, 2013, www.nytimes.com/2013/04/19/science/space/2-new-planets-are-most-earth-like-yet-scientists-say.html?pagewanted=all&_r=0.